Surgical Nursing in Practice

Alice Yip • Graeme Drummond Smith

Editors

Surgical Nursing in Practice

Perspectives on the Application of Clinical Expertise Towards Better Patient Care

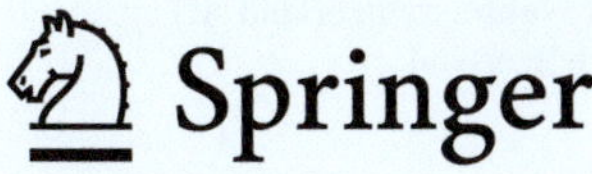 Springer

Editors
Alice Yip
School of Health Sciences
St. Francis University
Tseung Kwan O, Hong Kong

Graeme Drummond Smith
School of Health Sciences
St. Francis University
Tseung Kwan O, Hong Kong

ISBN 978-3-032-14728-8   ISBN 978-3-032-14729-5   (eBook)
https://doi.org/10.1007/978-3-032-14729-5

This Springer imprint is published by the registered company Springer Nature Switzerland AG
The registered company address is: Gewerbestrasse 11, 6330 Cham, Switzerland

If disposing of this product, please recycle the paper.

Foreword

This volume brings together a group of contributors to explore surgical nursing as both a clinical specialty and a developing field of professional knowledge. The work arose from the conviction that surgical nursing requires its own body of scholarship, one that acknowledges the technical, ethical, and cultural dimensions of care. While the book has been written within the Hong Kong context, its themes and insights have wider relevance for those engaged in the education and practice of surgery-related nursing.

The collection builds upon the *Caring Life-Course Theory*, which provides a unifying framework for understanding how care unfolds across time and circumstance. It recognizes that surgical interventions mark key turning points in people's lives, moments that test resilience, expose vulnerability, and call for professional skill and human presence in equal measure. The authors, representing a range of subspecialties, have sought to capture these realities through both conceptual discussion and clinical reflection.

The four sections, *Care Provision and Practice*; *Capability and Self-Care*; *Care Needs and Transitions*; and *Care Networks and Trajectories*, reflect the movement of the surgical patient's experience from admission to rehabilitation. This structure mirrors the continuity of care that surgical nurses increasingly provide, as practice expands beyond the operating theatre into preoperative preparation, community follow-up, and long-term support.

One of the strengths of the book lies in its attention to capability and professional formation. The sections on research, leadership, and simulation-based learning illustrate the intellectual maturity of the discipline. Surgical nursing is presented here as a field that is both practical and reflective, concerned not only with competence at the bedside but also with inquiry, evidence, and critical self-assessment. The contributors do not avoid the tensions inherent in modern health systems: resource constraints; workforce pressures; and the growing expectation that nurses act as both clinicians and educators.

Equally important are the chapters dealing with culture and transition. They remind us that surgery takes place within social and emotional worlds, not in isolation from them. The nursing response must therefore be attuned to beliefs, family structures, and cultural practices, ensuring that care is respectful as well as effective. This approach is particularly significant in Hong Kong and the wider Asian region, where patient diversity demands sensitivity and adaptability.

Professor of Nursing   Roger Watson
Saint Francis University
Tseung Kwan O, Hong Kong, China

Preface

It is with a profound sense of scholarly commitment and sincere dedication that we present this definitive work on advanced surgical nursing. This book is dedicated to the community of nursing specialists, educators, and scholars in caring science who are invested in the advancement of nursing practice in Asia. It is for those who seek to innovate and elevate patient care through a theoretically guided and humanistic lens.

The landscape of advanced surgical nursing is one of constant evolution, marked by rapid technological advancements and increasingly complex patient needs. In this high-stakes environment, it is easy to become interested in the technical aspects of care, focusing on the disease and the procedure. However, the essence of nursing, and indeed its enduring strength, lies in its holistic and human-centered approach. This book is a response to the critical need to anchor our sophisticated surgical nursing practices in a strong theoretical framework that honors the whole person.

To this end, we have chosen the Caring Life-Course Theory as the guiding theoretical compass for this scholarly discourse. The theory offers a comprehensive lens to view the patient's journey not as an isolated surgical event but as a significant life experience within the broader context of their individual life course. It calls on us to consider the patient's unique care biography, their personal history, and their network of relationships, which all play a crucial role in their health and well-being. By understanding the interplay of these factors, advanced practice nurses can provide care that is not only clinically excellent but also deeply compassionate and respectful of the patient's dignity.

This book is structured into four thematic sections, each designed to build upon the last, guiding the reader from the tangible applications of practice to the broader, long-term perspectives of patient care trajectories.

Our exploration begins with the core of our profession in *Part I: Care Provision and Practice*. This section grounds our discussion in the direct, specialized application of advanced nursing in diverse surgical settings. Chapters here provide exemplars of excellence, detailing the work of ophthalmic nurses caring for patients with cataracts, the critical role of neurosurgical nursing for patients undergoing neurosurgeries, the specialized environment of theatre nursing within operating theatres, and the compassionate practice of pediatric nursing for children with stoma-related problems. These contributions delineate the noticeable impact of dedicated, hands-on care.

From this foundation, we move to *Part II: Capability and Self-Care*. This section examines the professional architecture that supports and empowers the advanced surgical nurse. It explores the symbiotic relationship between research and education in surgical nursing, offers leadership perspectives on achieving surgical expertise, and presents innovative approaches to simulation education and practice. A key chapter on urological nursing expertise demonstrates how new techniques and approaches directly enhance patient outcomes, illustrating the vital link between a nurse's capability and the patient's well-being.

Part III: Care Needs and Transitions shifts the focus to the patient's experiential journey, particularly during critical and often vulnerable life transitions. This section explores the nuanced and deeply human aspects of nursing. We explore how colorectal nursing specialists use advanced strategies to bridge communication and cultural gaps when caring for patients with colorectal cancer in Chinese communities. Further chapters illuminate how breast nursing specialists deliver compassionate care to patients with breast cancer and share the profound experiences of organ donation coordinators in Hong Kong, highlighting the nurse's role in navigating pivotal life moments.

Finally, *Part IV: Care Networks and Trajectories* broadens our lens to consider the long-term management and holistic journey of the patient, extending far beyond the immediate surgical event. This section addresses the continuity of care and the networks that sustain it. Chapters feature the comprehensive approach of burn nursing specialists in advancing burn care and rehabilitation, discussions by cardiothoracic nursing specialists on advancements in chest drainage systems for post-surgical patients, and the vital work of enterostomal therapy nursing specialists in enhancing the long-term quality of life for patients with a stoma.

This text endeavors to provide a comprehensive exploration of advanced surgical nursing through the prism of the Caring Life-Course Theory. It is our sincere hope that this work will serve as an invaluable resource for nursing specialists seeking to enhance their clinical practice, for educators shaping the next generation of nursing leaders, and for scholars dedicated to advancing the scientific underpinnings of our profession. We believe that by embracing a theoretical framework that champions a holistic and patient-centered approach, we can collectively elevate the standard of care and reaffirm the profound and ongoing value of nursing in the surgical arena and beyond.

<table>
<tr><td>Tseung Kwan O, Hong Kong, China</td><td>Alice Yip</td></tr>
<tr><td>Tseung Kwan O, Hong Kong, China</td><td>Graeme Drummond Smith</td></tr>
</table>

Acknowledgments

As the editor of this book, it is my distinct honor to articulate a deep and sincere gratitude to the community of nursing specialists and scholars whose collective wisdom forms the very foundation of this book. The completion of this scholarly endeavor, aimed at charting the course of advanced surgical nursing, represents the confluence of numerous expert voices and a shared, unwavering dedication to the science and art of caring.

My most profound appreciation is extended to the esteemed nursing specialists and distinguished scholars who have so generously contributed their intellectual and experiential capital to these pages. They have done far more than simply author chapters; they have opened a window into the intricate, demanding realities of their clinical worlds. With remarkable truthfulness and scholarly precision, they have shared narratives of practice imbued with wisdom that can only be forged in the crucible of direct patient care. Their contributions move beyond the abstract, providing authentic, situated perspectives on the challenges and triumphs of caring for patients navigating complex surgical journeys. It is through these real-world accounts that the theoretical underpinnings of our work find their most powerful expression.

This book is uniquely enriched by its grounding in the Asian context. In this regard, a particular debt of gratitude is owed to the esteemed Fellows of the Hong Kong College of Surgical Nursing and all contributing nursing experts who graciously shared their valuable information. They have masterfully articulated the nuances of applying advanced nursing principles within our region's specific healthcare systems, diverse cultural tapestries, and unique patient populations. Their insights are invaluable, offering a perspective that is both globally relevant and locally sensitive. In sharing their clinical experiences, they are actively updating and refining our collective understanding of advanced nursing practice, ensuring it remains dynamic, responsive, and attuned to the communities we serve.

It has been a profound privilege to combine and present such a remarkable collection of expertise. This book stands as a testament to the collaborative spirit, clinical excellence, and deep-seated compassion of its contributors. For their partnership in this significant undertaking, and for their tireless commitment to advancing our profession and enhancing patient care, I am sincerely and deeply grateful.

Dr. Alice Yip

I wish to extend my sincere appreciation to the academic and clinical colleagues in Hong Kong, whose scholarly contributions have been instrumental in the development of this surgical nursing textbook. I am also grateful to the surgical nursing professionals and multidisciplinary healthcare teams around the world, whose appreciation and application of research, evidence-based practice, and commitment to excellence have provided a solid foundation for the material presented. In particular, I would like to extend my sincere gratitude to Dr. Alice Yip for her leadership on this textbook. Her scholarly contributions to this textbook and her dedication to advancing surgical nursing knowledge in Hong Kong have greatly enhanced both the content and academic rigor of this work. Finally, I wish to express my heartfelt gratitude to Maggie, Nathaniel, and Natalie for their unwavering support and understanding in the preparation of this text.

Professor Graeme Drummond Smith

Contents

Part I

Care Provision and Practice

The Integral Role of Ophthalmic Nurses in Preoperative Assessment and Management for Cataract Surgery Patients

1

Yee-Sheung Christina Tsang and Alice Yip

Introduction

Age-related cataracts are a major global cause of visual impairment, especially among older adults (Cicinelli et al. 2023; Steinmetz et al. 2021; Vision Loss Expert Group of the Global Burden of Disease Study 2024). Cataract surgery demonstrably enhances visual function, consequently improving the patient's quality of life (Wang et al. 2024). Contemporary advancements in surgical techniques, particularly phacoemulsification (small incision cataract surgery), have facilitated the widespread adoption of day-case procedures of most patients (Leffler et al. 2020; Narayan et al. 2023).

Hong Kong is experiencing a demographic shift toward an aging population (Census and Statistics Department, HKSAR 2023). Of its approximately 7.5 million citizens, 1.6 million individuals aged 65 and older are currently awaiting cataract surgery. This considerable waiting list highlights the increasing demand for ophthalmological services within the context of Hong Kong's aging demographic (Lo 2024). Data from the Hospital Authority indicate that the maximum waiting time for cataract surgery is currently 52 months (Hospital Authority 2025). This chapter explores the clinical presentation of cataracts, emphasizing the essential role of nursing care. It considers the impact of cataracts on quality of life and details the function of nurse-led preoperative assessment clinics, highlighting their holistic approach. The chapter covers care plan implementation, outcome evaluation, and

Y.-S. C. Tsang (✉)
Advanced Practice Nurse, Department of Ophthalmology and Visual Sciences, Prince of Wales Hospital, Shatin, HKSAR, China
e-mail: tys024@ha.org.hk

A. Yip
School of Health Sciences, St. Francis University,
Tseung Kwan O, Hong Kong
e-mail: khyip@sfu.edu.hk

3

pre- and postoperative carer, including patient education. Finally, it reviews current treatment modalities, aiming to provide a comprehensive understanding of cataracts and the importance of nursing in optimizing patient outcomes.

Quality of Life in Patients with Cataracts

Cataracts significantly impact the quality of life for older adults, extending beyond mere visual impairment (Harsi et al. 2023; Wang et al. 2024). The presence of cataracts increases the risk of falls, a serious concern in these people (Schlenker et al. 2018). This elevated risk is multifactorial, with visual impairment playing a crucial role. Specifically, uncorrected refractive errors associated with cataracts negatively affect balance and depth perception (Hashemi et al. 2023; Naël et al. 2019; Schlenker et al. 2018). Reduced contrast sensitivity, glare, and declined visual acuity (VA) contribute to difficulties in navigating the environment, judging distances, and perceiving changes in sphere, all of which raise fall risk (Jin et al. 2024). Furthermore, the visual limitations urged by cataracts can lead to social isolation, depression, and a decrease in overall well-being (Dhawale and Tidake 2024; Wang et al. 2024). Therefore, timely cataract intervention is critical not only for restoring visual function but also for reducing the broader negative impacts on older adults' quality of life, independence, and overall health (Wang et al. 2024).

Preoperative Assessment Clinic

Preoperative assessment clinics (PAOCs) are crucial for enhancing ophthalmological surgical services, particularly within the public sectors in Hong Kong (Hospital Authority). These ophthalmic nurse clinics address increasing demands for procedures like cataract surgery by streamlining patient evaluation and preparation through a one-stop, specialized, multidisciplinary approach. Ophthalmic nurses conduct comprehensive assessments, including patient education, optimizing surgical readiness and minimizing cancellations (Tung Wah Eastern Hospital 2021; Zhang and Cao 2024). This model provides focused preoperative care for patients listed for elective cataract surgery. Furthermore, patients receive telephone reminders regarding their surgical appointments to ensure smooth operation scheduling and reduce the likelihood of missed appointments or delays. This approach lessens the burden on ophthalmologists, shortens waiting lists, and improves patient satisfaction. By implementing standardized protocols and risk class, these clinics ensure high-quality, efficient care, finally leading to better patient outcomes and a more effective healthcare system (Sharbini et al. 2025; Zhang and Cao 2024).

In Hong Kong, the Hospital Authority offers the Post-Registration Certification Course (PRCC) in Ophthalmic Nursing, an advanced professional development program for nurse specializing in ophthalmology. Registered nurses with a minimum of 5 years of experience in ophthalmic nursing and holding the PRCC are designated as ophthalmic nurses. Patients scheduled for elective cataract surgery within the public sectors (eye centers) are placed on a waiting list by ophthalmologists and are required to undergo a preoperative assessment between 2 and 8 weeks prior to the procedure. This assessment involves a collaborative approach between ophthalmologists and ophthalmic nurses, who jointly conduct health assessments and relevant investigations (Zhang and Cao 2024). This collaborative process facilitates the early identification of potential risk factors, including uncontrolled hypertension, poorly managed diabetes mellitus, cardiac conditions, recent stroke, current medications (e.g., anticoagulants), respiratory diseases, infectious diseases, hearing impairment, and mental illness (Sharbini et al. 2024).

Holistic Patient Assessment

A holistic approach to ocular assessment prioritizes the patient's comprehensive experience, moving beyond a diagnosis-centric model (Lockey and Hassan 2009; Stewart et al. 2024). Assessment should be patient-centered to foster independence and enhance quality of life (Assi et al. 2021; Kaštelan et al. 2024). This comprehensive ocular assessment utilizes techniques, such as slit-lamp biomicroscopy, VA measurements, and intraocular pressure (IOP) evaluations (Munteanu et al. 2024; Upadhyaya et al. 2022; Yazu et al. 2020). Holistic ocular assessment incorporates different techniques. Slit-lamp biomicroscopy applies a high-intensity light source and microscope to examine anterior eye structures, including the eyelids, cornea, conjunctiva, iris, lens, and anterior chamber, facilitating detailed assessment for abnormalities. VA measurements, often applying standardized charts with progressively smaller optotypes, assess the clarity of vision at varying distances. Finally, IOP evaluations, frequently conducted via tonometry, calculate fluid pressure within the eye, as evaluated IOP is a primary risk factor for glaucoma and potential optic nerve damage.

Cataract surgery and its subsequent management involve a multifaceted, multiprofessional approach involving ophthalmologists, optometrists, dispensing opticians, nurses, and technicians. Each professional provides specialized expertise and shares essential information to comprehensively plan, perform, and evaluate the outcome of each procedure. This collaborative, interdisciplinary model strengthens the connection between primary and secondary care, ensuring comprehensive patient care (Baker et al. 2016). Ophthalmic nurses play a particularly required role in this process, providing essential support and expertise throughout the patient's surgical journey. Their contributions extend beyond basic care to contain advanced assessment techniques, such as slit-lamp biomicroscopy (Sharbini et al. 2024). Furthermore, ophthalmic nurses conduct fundamental diagnostic tests, including VA measurements, IOP assessments, and auto-refraction, contributing significantly to a comprehensive understanding of the patient's ocular health (Sharbini et al. 2024). This holistic approach, with nursing care as a cornerstone, enhances patient outcomes and secures the delivery of high-quality, patient-centered care throughout the cataract management process. The specialized skills and knowledge base of ophthalmic nurses are integral to effective preoperative education, postoperative care, and ongoing monitoring, eventually contributing to enhanced patient satisfaction and visual rehabilitation (Sharbini et al. 2024).

Implementation of a Nursing Care Plan

Ophthalmic nurses act a critical role in the preoperative assessment and management of patients undergoing cataract surgery. Proactive identification of ocular risk factors, such as blepharitis and chalazion, is essential, allowing the implementation of a tailored nursing care plan to monitor and address the patient's specific ocular needs (Alofi et al. 2024). This plan helps to continue assessment, targeted interventions, and patient education. Furthermore, the ophthalmic nurse plays a crucial role in estimating the patient's overall health status. If a patient presents with unstable medical conditions, such as uncontrolled hypertension, which could lead to a risk during surgery, the nurse facilitates referral back to the patient's primary care physician or relevant specialist in out-patient department. This secures appropriate medical optimization prior to cataract surgery. Moreover, patients who need additional support or specialized care are proactively referred to allied healthcare professionals, assisting early intervention and comprehensive management (Annoh et al. 2019). This collaborative approach, with the ophthalmic nurse as a central coordinator, ensures patient safety and optimizes surgical outcomes. In the Hong Kong healthcare context, this integrated approach is particularly significant, ensuring patients receive comprehensive care and acquire to the necessary medical expertise before undergoing cataract surgery.

Checking Cataract Surgery Results: Getting Patients Ready

Following optimization of the patient's systemic health and ocular status, the ophthalmic nurse handles a comprehensive assessment to assess the potential outcomes of cataract surgery and the patient's readiness for the procedure. This evaluation requires a holistic approach, regarding the patient's physical, psychological, and social well-being (Assi et al. 2021; Dhawale and Tidake 2024; Wang et al. 2024). Factors considered include the patient's understanding of the procedure, expectations for anxiety levels, visual improvement, and support systems. Physical assessment comprises VA measurements, biomicroscopy to evaluate the ocular structures, and relevant diagnostic tests, such as A-scan biometry for intraocular lens power calculation (Shammas and Shammas 2024). Social factors, such as living environments, caregiver availability, and access to transportation, are also taught to arrange appropriate postoperative care (Błachnio et al. 2024). Based on this comprehensive assessment, the ophthalmic nurse collaborates with the ophthalmologist and the patient (and their caregiver, if applicable) to determine the optimal timing for cataract surgery and make the essential arrangements for the procedure. This patient-centered approach makes sure that the surgery is operated when the patient is ideally prepared, both physically and psychologically, maximizing the likelihood of a successful outcome (Holch et al. 2020).

Patient Education: Empowering Patients for Cataract Surgery

Preoperative patient education is vital for empowering patients to make informed decisions regarding their care and to secure their active participation in postoperative self-management (Stanford 2023; Wisely et al. 2020). An individualized approach should be adopted when determining the most essential mode of patient education. For instance, transferring information through videos played in the cataract pre-assessment clinic can be a valuable tool for some patients (Wisely et al. 2020). Alternatively, as suggested by some studies, face-to-face preoperative education can be particularly successful in lessening anxiety levels in individuals undergoing cataract surgery (Kumar et al. 2023; Vasquez-Perez and Liu 2021). The optimal approach should be resolved through a thorough assessment carried out during the nurse-patient interaction, regarding individual patient needs, learning preferences, and potential barriers to understanding. This personalized approach ensures that the information delivered is tailored to each patient, enhancing its effectiveness and promoting successful postoperative outcomes.

Preoperative Care

The primary objective of cataract surgery is to optimize the patient's VA. Following the procedure, patients can anticipate a significant improvement in both near and distance vision, enhancing their overall functional vision and quality of life (Marcos et al. 2021).

Patient Education

Preoperative cataract surgery education is vital and integral, including a detailed explanation of the procedure (steps, anesthesia, duration), expected recovery (discomfort, timeframe, visual outcomes), and lifestyle modifications (avoiding strenuous activities, eye rubbing, and dust/water exposure) (Choi and Greenberg 2018; Cnaany et al. 2024). Clear instructions regarding postoperative medications, particularly eye drops, are important. Encouraging questions promotes a collaborative approach, safeguard patients are well-informed and prepared, leading to active recovery participation and positive surgical experience.

Comfort Measures

Implementing comfort measures are needed to alleviate patient anxiety and address concerns regarding cataract surgery. These measures may comprise clear and empathetic communication, answering questions thoroughly, and providing a calm and supportive atmosphere. Furthermore, preoperative assessment should include recording the

International Normalized Ratio (INR) for patients on warfarin therapy to evaluate coagulation status (Makuloluwa et al. 2019). A comprehensive mobility and fall risk assessment should also be performed to identify potential postoperative complications and implement preventative strategies. Securing valid informed consent, enclosing a thorough explanation of the procedure, risk, and benefits, is vital. Finally integrating health promotion principles, such as encouraging patients on healthy lifestyle choices, contributes to overall well-being and positive surgical outcomes (Choi and Greenberg 2018; Cnaany et al. 2024).

Postoperative Care

Postoperative care after cataract surgery is critical for optimal vision recovery and preventing complications (Webber et al. 2020). This care consists of monitoring VA and implementing safety measures to secure the patient's eye during the healing process.

Monitoring VA

Post-cataract surgery, regular VA assessments applying standardized charts are necessary for monitoring recovery and detecting complications, such as inflammation, infection, or posterior capsule opacification (Webber et al. 2020). These assessments, conducted at prescribed intervals, inhibit timely intervention and optimize visual outcomes.

Safety Measures

Maintaining a safe environment for cataract surgery is vital, requiring comprehensive risk management and infection prevention for patients and staff—a need emphasized by public crises like the COVID-19 pandemic (Webber et al. 2020; Yip et al. 2025; Zhang et al. 2022). This involves decreasing fall risks and protecting the operated eye from accidental trauma. Furthermore, optimizing visual function needs comprehensive support, assisting patients in adapting to their improved, yet potentially altered, vision (Zhang et al. 2022). This adaptation process may include guidance on utilizing prescribed eye drops, controlling temporary visual disturbances such as glare or halos, and adjusting to changes in depth perception. The decision regarding overnight hospitalization is determined by factors such as the complexity of the surgical procedure, preexisting medical conditions, the patient's ability to carry out activities of daily living, and the availability of adequate support at home. Patients who live alone, lack sufficient support, or experience difficulties with daily activities may need hospitalization to guarantee proper postoperative care and minimize potential complications.

Conclusion

Sight-limiting cataracts significantly impact the physical and psychological well-being of older adults, emphasizing the critical need for effective and accessible cataract services. POACs represent a unique and promising approach to address the expected rise in demand for pre- and postoperative cataract surgery assessments. Within these clinics, advanced practice ophthalmic nurses can develop, delivering holistic, patient-centered care and demonstrably enhancing patient outcomes. By broadening the scope of practice for these highly skilled nurses, healthcare systems can optimize resource utilization and secure timely access to high-quality care. Future research and planning should focus on exploring the full potential of these resources and developing strategies to accomplish optimal patient outcomes in the emerging landscape of cataract care.

References

Alofi RM, Alrohaily LS, Alharthi NN, Almouteri MM, Almouteri M (2024) Ocular manifestations in seborrheic dermatitis epidemiology, clinical features, and management: a comprehensive review. Cureus 16(9). https://doi.org/10.7759/cureus.70335

Annoh R, Patel S, Beck D, Ellis H, Dhillon B, Sanders R (2019) Digital ophthalmology in Scotland: benefits to patient care and education. Clin Ophthalmol (Auckland, NZ) 13:277. https://doi.org/10.2147/OPTH.S185186

Assi L, Chamseddine F, Ibrahim P, Sabbagh H, Rosman L, Congdon N, Evans J, Ramke J, Kuper H, Burton MJ, Ehrlich JR, Swenor BK (2021) A global assessment of eye health and quality of life: a systematic review of systematic reviews. JAMA Ophthalmol 139(5):526–541. https://doi.org/10.1001/jamaophthalmol.2021.0146

Baker H, Ratnarajan G, Harper RA, Edgar DF, Lawrenson JG (2016) Effectiveness of UK optometric enhanced eye care services: a realist review of the literature. Ophthalmic Physiol Opt 36(5):545–557. https://doi.org/10.1111/opo.12312

Błachnio K, Dusińska A, Szymonik J, Juzwiszyn J, Bestecka M, Chabowski M (2024) Quality of life after cataract surgery. J Clin Med 13(17):5209. https://doi.org/10.3390/jcm13175209

Census and Statistics Department, The Government of the Hong Kong Special Administrative Region (HKSAR) (2023) Hong Kong population projections for 2022 to 2046. The Government of the Hong Kong Special Administrative Region. Online available: https://www.censtatd.gov.hk/en/EIndexbySubject.html?scode=190&pcode=FA100061. Accessed on 30 June 2025

Choi AR, Greenberg PB (2018) Patient education strategies in cataract surgery: a systematic review. J Evid Based Med 11(2):71–82. https://doi.org/10.1111/jebm.12297

Cicinelli MV, Buchan JC, Nicholson M, Varadaraj V, Khanna RC (2023) Cataracts. Lancet 401(10374):377–389. https://doi.org/10.1016/S0140-6736(22)01839-6

Cnaany Y, Goldstein A, Lavy I, Halpert M, Chowers I, Ben-Eli H (2024) Ophthalmology residents' experience in cataract surgery: preoperative risk factors, intraoperative complications, and surgical outcomes. Ophthalmol Therapy 13(6):1783–1798. https://doi.org/10.1007/s40123-024-00947-6

Dhawale KK, Tidake P (2024) Cataract surgery and mental health: a comprehensive review on outcomes in the elderly. Cureus 16(7). https://doi.org/10.7759/cureus.65469

Harsi EE, Benksim A, Kasmaoui FE, Cherkaoui M (2023) Factors associated with quality of life among older adults with cataract. NPG Neurologie-Psychiatrie-Gériatrie 23(137):306–314. https://doi.org/10.1016/j.npg.2023.05.008

Hashemi A, Khabazkhoob M, Hashemi H (2023) High prevalence of refractive errors in an elderly population; a public health issue. BMC Ophthalmol 23(1):38. https://doi.org/10.1186/s12886-023-02791-x

Holch P, Absolom K, Brooke C, Wang X (2020) Advances in patient reported outcomes: integration and innovation. J Patient Report Outcomes 4(Suppl 1):28. https://doi.org/10.1186/s41687-020-00193-x

Hospital Authority (2025) Elective cataract surgery. Hospital Authority. Online available: https://www.ha.org.hk/visitor/ha_visitor_index.asp?Content_ID=214184&Lang=ENG&Dimension=10. Accessed on 30 June 2025

Jin H, Zhou Y, Stagg BC, Ehrlich JR (2024) Association between vision impairment and increased prevalence of falls in older US adults. J Am Geriatr Soc 72(5):1373–1383. https://doi.org/10.1111/jgs.18879

Kaštelan S, Pjevač N, Braš M, Đorđević V, Keleminić NP, Mezzich JE (2024) Person-centered care in ophthalmology: current knowledge and perspectives. Croat Med J 65(2):156. https://doi.org/10.3325/cmj.2024.65.156

Kumar SP, Vishwakarma P, Ranpise D, Chavan S, Krishnan R, Kurian E, Team MFV (2023) A multisite longitudinal investigation of psychological outcomes following cataract surgery in India. Indian J Psychol Med 45(6):598–609. https://doi.org/10.1177/02537176231172300

Leffler CT, Klebanov A, Samara WA, Grzybowski A (2020) The history of cataract surgery: from couching to phacoemulsification. Ann Transl Med 8(22):1551. https://doi.org/10.21037/atm-2019-rcs-04

Lo CM (2024) LCQ6: cataract surgeries. The Government of the Hong Kong Special Administrative Region. Online available: https://www.info.gov.hk/gia/general/202411/20/P2024112000464.htm. Accessed on 30 June 2025

Lockey J, Hassan MU (2009) Holistic approach to pre-operative assessment for cataract patients. Br J Nurs 18(5):323–327. https://doi.org/10.12968/bjon.2009.18.5.40547

Makuloluwa AK, Tiew S, Briggs M (2019) Peri-operative management of ophthalmic patients on anti-thrombotic agents: a literature review. Eye 33(7):1044–1059. https://doi.org/10.1038/s41433-019-0382-6

Marcos S, Martinez-Enriquez E, Vinas M, de Castro A, Dorronsoro C, Bang SP, Yoon G, Artal P (2021) Simulating outcomes of cataract surgery: important advances in ophthalmology. Annu Rev Biomed Eng 23(1):277–306. https://doi.org/10.1146/annurev-bioeng-082420-035827

Munteanu M, Mocanu V, Preda A (2024) Ophthalmological pathology and medical and surgical management in eye disease cataract. In: Clinical ophthalmology: a guide to diagnosis and treatment. Springer Nature Switzerland, Cham, pp 225–247. https://doi.org/10.1007/978-3-031-68453-1_9

Naël V, Moreau G, Monfermé S, Cougnard-Grégoire A, Scherlen AC, Arleo A, Korobelnik J, Delcourt C, Helmer C (2019) Prevalence and associated factors of uncorrected refractive error in older adults in a population-based study in France. JAMA Ophthalmol 137(1):3–11. https://doi.org/10.1001/jamaophthalmol.2018.4229

Narayan A, Evans JR, O'Brart D, Bunce C, Gore DM, Day AC (2023) Laser-assisted cataract surgery versus standard ultrasound phacoemulsification cataract surgery. Cochrane Database Syst Rev 6. https://doi.org/10.1002/14651858.CD010735.pub3

Schlenker MB, Thiruchelvam D, Redelmeier DA (2018) Association of cataract surgery with traffic crashes. JAMA Ophthalmol 136(9):998–1007. https://doi.org/10.1001/jamaophthalmol.2018.2510

Shammas MC, Shammas HJ (2024) The A-scan biometer. In: Intraocular lens calculations. Springer International Publishing, Cham, pp 289–296. https://doi.org/10.1007/978-3-031-50666-6_16

Sharbini, S., Abdul-Mumin, K. H., & McKenna, L. (2025). Ophthalmic care education and training in nursing: A scoping review. Nurse Education Today, 144, 106484. https://doi.org/10.1016/j.nedt.2024.106484

Stanford P (2023) Cataracts: the essentials for patient care. Br J Community Nurs 28(5):230–236. https://doi.org/10.12968/bjcn.2023.28.5.230

Steinmetz JD, Bourne RR, Briant PS, Flaxman SR, Taylor HR, Jonas JB et al (2021) Causes of blindness and vision impairment in 2020 and trends over 30 years, and prevalence of avoidable blindness in relation to VISION 2020: the right to sight: an analysis for the global burden of disease study. Lancet Glob Health 9(2):e144–e160. https://doi.org/10.1016/S2214-109X(20)30489-7

Stewart M, Brown JB, Weston WW, Freeman T, Ryan BL, McWilliam CL, McWhinney IR (2024) Patient-centered medicine: transforming the clinical method. CRC Press, Boca Raton

Tung Wah Eastern Hospital (2021) Hospital services: nurse clinic (cataract surgery). Hospital Authority. Online available: https://www.ha.org.hk/tweh/eng/services/02/02d_frame.htm. Accessed on 30 June 2025

Upadhyaya S, Agarwal A, Rengaraj V, Srinivasan K, Newman Casey PA, Schehlein E (2022) Validation of a portable, non-mydriatic fundus camera compared to gold standard dilated fundus examination using slit lamp biomicroscopy for assessing the optic disc for glaucoma. Eye 36(2):441–447. https://doi.org/10.1038/s41433-021-01485-2

Vasquez-Perez A, Liu C (2021) What do cataract patients want? In: Cataract surgery: pearls and techniques. Springer, Cham, pp 1–12. https://doi.org/10.1007/978-3-030-38234-6_1

Vision Loss Expert Group of the Global Burden of Disease Study (2024) Global estimates on the number of people blind or visually impaired by cataract: a meta-analysis from 2000 to 2020. Eye 38(11):2156. https://doi.org/10.1038/s41433-024-02961-1

Wang S, Du Z, Lai C, Seth I, Wang Y, Huang Y, Fang Y, Liao H, Hu Y, Yu H, Zhang X (2024) The association between cataract surgery and mental health in older adults: a review. Int J Surg 110(4):2300–2312. https://doi.org/10.1097/JS9.0000000000001105

Webber KJ, Fylan F, Wood JM, Elliott DB (2020) Experiences following cataract surgery–patient perspectives. Ophthalmic Physiol Opt 40(5):540–548. https://doi.org/10.1111/opo.12709

Wisely CE, Robbins CB, Stinnett S, Kim T, Vann RR, Gupta PK (2020) Impact of preoperative video education for cataract surgery on patient learning outcomes. Clin Ophthalmol 14:1365–1371. https://doi.org/10.2147/OPTH.S248080

Yazu H, Shimizu E, Okuyama S, Katahira T, Aketa N, Yokoiwa R, Sato Y, Ogawa Y, Fujishima H (2020) Evaluation of nuclear cataract with smartphone-attachable slit-lamp device. Diagnostics 10(8):576. https://doi.org/10.3390/diagnostics10080576

Yip A, Yip J, Tsui Z, Yip CH, Lung HL, Shit KY, Yip R (2025) The impact of COVID on healthcare services, risk management, and infection prevention in surgical settings: a qualitative study. Healthcare 13:579. https://doi.org/10.3390/healthcare13060579

Zhang Y, Cao N (2024) Integrating nurse-led interventions in ophthalmology care: a systematic review. J Nurs Care Qual 39(4):E61–E67. https://doi.org/10.1097/NCQ.0000000000000788

Zhang JH, Ramke J, Lee CN, Gordon I, Safi S, Lingham G, Evans JR, Keel S (2022) A systematic review of clinical practice guidelines for cataract: evidence to support the development of the WHO package of eye care interventions. Vision 6(2):36. https://doi.org/10.3390/vision6020036

Investigating the Crucial Function and Growth of Specialized Nursing Services in Advancing Neurosurgical Patient Care: Understandings and Consequences

Kwun-Lin Man and Alice Yip

Introduction

The global landscape of neurosurgical care is undergoing a paradigm shift, precipitated by rapid technological advancements and the increasing complexity of patient pathophysiology. A corresponding evolution in the scope of nursing practice is not merely an adjunct to this transformation but a fundamental prerequisite for delivery safe and effective patient care. The emergence of specialty nursing services within neurosurgery is illustrated by a recent initiative in Hong Kong, which provides an applicable exemplar of this trend for this discussion (Hospital Authority, Strategy and Planning Division 2016). The establishment of this service provides a critical case study for examining the opportunities and challenges inherent in formalizing an expanded nursing role within a high-acuity medical specialty.

A cornerstone of this service model is the establishment of the neurosurgical nurse clinic, a strategic initiative that formalizes the expanded scope of practice (Pugh et al. 2022). These clinics provide a structured framework for delivering a continuum of specialized healthcare interventions, thereby amplifying the contribution of the nursing team. The service operates on a collaborative model, integrating the distinct expertise of nursing consultants, advanced practice nurses, and registered nurses. This integrated team of professionals works in synergy to provide comprehensive and specialized nursing care for neurosurgical patients within the public sector in Hong Kong.

K.-L. Man (✉)
Hong Kong College of Surgical Nursing, Kowloon, HKSAR, China
e-mail: mankl@ha.org.hk

A. Yip
School of Health Sciences, St. Francis University,
Tseung Kwan O, Hong Kong
e-mail: khyip@sfu.edu.hk

Hospital Authority facilities an advanced practice training program in neuroscience nursing, elevating the clinical proficiency of its specialist team. This program extends beyond foundational neuroscience qualifications to cultivate a sophisticated portfolio of advanced technical competencies (Institute of Advanced Nursing Studies 2024). This includes proficiency in transcranial Doppler monitoring, intra-operative neurophysiological monitoring (IONM), and electroencephalography (EEG). Skills are indispensable for the real-time assessment and management of patients with complex neurological pathologies. The practice of these nurse specialists transcends traditional departmental boundaries, with their roles integrated into ambulatory care, inpatient ward, and the operating theater (HOSPITAL AUTHORITY, STRATEGY AND PLANNING DIVISION 2016).

Furthermore, their integral involvement in many clinical activities, such as grand rounds, preoperative meetings, and multidisciplinary treatments planning meetings, is fundamental to fostering interdisciplinary synergy in public sector. This collaboration practice model is designed to optimize patient safety, rationalize care pathways, and ultimately elevate the standard of neurosurgical care and patient outcomes within the region (Lee et al. 2021).

The Multifaceted Role of the Neurosurgical Nurse Specialist Team

The fundamental function of the neurosurgical nurse specialist team is rooted in deep coordination and collaboration with the broader multidisciplinary team. This interdisciplinary synergy fosters a dynamic and evolving process of care, which is essential for adeptly addressing the complex and often fluctuating needs of both patients and their families. They serve as a pivotal resource, providing patients and their families with critical health-related information, navigating them toward community support systems, and acting as advocates. This includes targeted health education and health promotion, empowering patients to become active participants in their own care. Operationally, the team's responsibilities span the patient journey; oversee care throughout hospitalization and arrange comprehensive discharge plans well in advance of the patient's discharge (Cartwright and Kennedy 2025). By managing these clinical pathways and considering the underlying clinic logistics, the nursing team ensures the delivery of a seamless and comprehensive specialty nurse service.

From Case Management to Quantifiable Outcomes: The Impact of the Nurse-Led Service

The nurse-led clinic in neurosurgery is a sophisticated and integrated model of care, providing continuous and holistic support to patients throughout their entire perioperative journey. This service functions as the central pillar of a patient-centered approach, shifting from task-oriented duties to comprehensive case management that demonstrably enhances clinical outcomes and healthcare system efficiency.

The service's scope begins with patient assessment, which includes detailed health histories, a full spectrum of neurosurgical, cognitive, and sensory evaluation, and risk stratification, including vision, smell, and taste test. This foundational workup creates a personalized baseline that informs all subsequent care. A core function is proactive medication management, where nurses monitor compliance, provide critical education on adherence and side effects, and manage therapeutic drug levels for medications like anticonvulsants and hormonal profile (Miao et al. 2023; Shady et al. 2025). Acting as central case managers for complex procedures including spine, brain, functional, and neuro-endovascular surgeries, these specialist nurses arrange necessary investigations, facilitate timely multidisciplinary referrals, and are vital participants in preoperative planning meetings, where they contribute an essential nursing perspective (Shady et al. 2025). Their role extends to addressing the patients' psychosocial state, identifying barriers to recovery, and providing reassurance to diminish the profound anxiety associated with neurosurgery (Miao et al. 2023; Oteri et al. 2021). Postoperatively, they deliver expert wound and implant management, cautiously detect complications, and ensure continuity of care.

The specific nursing management for a patient undergoing an awake craniotomy serves as a powerful exemplar of this model's depth (Mofatteh et al. 2023). Here, patient involvement is paramount, and the nurse's primary goal is to optimize emotional readiness and cooperation. This intensive process begins in the clinic with a detailed preoperative interview designed to build a strong rapport and trusting relationship. The nurse provides comprehensive education on all phases of care, from skin preparation to the admission process. They conduct baseline neurological and language assessments, then actively teach and rehearse the specific motor and cognitive tasks the patient must perform during the operation for brain mapping (Ibrahim et al. 2025; Roland et al. 2021).

The COVID-19 pandemic reshaped presurgical coordination, where nurses arrange assessments such as computed tomography (CT scan), magnetic resonance imaging (MRI) (for brain), functional MRI (for motor, speech mapping), and diffusion tensor imaging (DTI) with a multidisciplinary team, like anesthesiologists, clinical psychologists, physiotherapists, and occupational therapists. This crisis necessitated new risk management and infection prevention strategies in surgical settings, including rigorous patient screening, enhanced personal protective equipment (PPE), and rescheduled services to mitigate viral transmission (Yip et al. 2025). These measures profoundly impacted healthcare delivery, ensuring patient and staff safety while navigating the challenges of a public health emergency, often altering traditional presurgery visits (Shady et al. 2025; Cartwright and Kennedy 2025). Intraoperatively, the nurse becomes the patient's dedicated advocate and anchor. They provide highly personalized, one-on-one care, ensuring the patient's dignity is maintained while constantly assessing their needs for comfort, such as managing dry mouth or pain (Errico and Luoma 2023; Lindlöf et al. 2024). They are often a continuous stream of communication, informing the patient of progress to resolve anxiety. During the critical brain mapping procedure, the nurses guide the patient through the prerehearsal tasks, assist the surgical team with neurophysiological monitoring, and meticulously document responses to ensure the preservation of vital brain function.

The advantages of this comprehensive approach are validated by outstanding evaluation metrics. The service fosters a trusted relationship that improves patient understanding, reduces stress, and enhances compliance, leading to optimized clinical outcomes and more efficient discharge and rehabilitation planning (Guldager et al. 2022; Lindlöf et al. 2024). The success of this initiative is clearly demonstrated through exceptionally high levels of patient satisfaction and a noticeable trend toward shorter hospital stays, emphasizing its immense value to both patients and the public healthcare sector in Hong Kong.

The Emergence and Impact of Nurse-Led Intraoperative Neurophysiological Monitoring Services

Intraoperative Neurophysiological Monitoring

Intraoperative neurophysiological monitoring (IONM) represents a critical advancement in modern surgical practice, particularly within the complex field of neurosurgery. It is defined as the application electrophysiological monitoring techniques to assess the functional integrity of the central and peripheral nervous system during surgical procedures (Guzzi et al. 2024; Wilson Jr et al. 2023). The primary objective of IONM is to minimize the risk of iatrogenic neurological injury, thereby preserving neural function and enhancing patient outcomes (Wilson Jr et al. 2023). By providing real-time feedback on the status of neural pathways, IONM assists surgeons in navigating delicate structures, such as eloquent brain regions, spinal cord tracts, and peripheral nerves (Bianchi and Del Carro 2024; Guzzi et al. 2024). This practice has become indispensable in a variety of complex procedures, including brain and spinal tumor resections, epilepsy surgery, awake craniotomies, and neurovascular interventions (Alvarez et al. 2023; Bu et al. 2021; Guzzi et al. 2024).

While traditionally performed by neurophysiologists or technicians, an innovative and effective model of care has emerged: the nurse-led IONM service. This model influences the unique skill set of specialist nurses to provide a holistic, patient-centered approach that integrates technical expertise with comprehensive patient care throughout the surgical journey.

The Role of the Nurse Specialist Across the Perioperative Continuum

The effectiveness of a nurse-led IONM service is rooted in its continuous and integrated involvement across all phases of patient care: preoperative, intraoperative, and postoperative.

Preoperative Phase: Planning and Preparation

The foundation for successful IONM is laid before the patient enters the operating theater. In the preoperative phase, the nurse specialist conducts a thorough assessment of the patient's baseline neurological status (Goonasekera and Smith 2021). A key aspect of this phase is patient education; the nurse specialist explains the IONM procedure, helping to alleviate patient fear and anxiety while establishing a relationship build on trust (Goonasekera and Smith 2021; Lindlöf et al. 2024; Zentner et al. 2024).

Crucially, the nurse specialist collaborates closely with neurosurgeons, anesthesiologists, and other healthcare professionals in a preoperative meeting. This multidisciplinary approach ensures that a specific, individualized monitoring plan is developed for each patient (Lindlöf et al. 2024). This plan outlines the specific multi-modalities to be used, such as EEG, electrocorticography (ECoG), transcranial electrical motor evoked potentials (TCeMEP), or D-waves monitoring (Kumar et al. 2021). Furthermore, the nurse is responsible for the early setup and rigorous checking of all IONM equipment, confirming its proper function to guarantee patient safety and procedural efficacy.

Intraoperative Phase: Attentiveness and Real-Time Intervention

During the surgical procedure, the nurse specialist's role is highly dynamic and critical. Responsibilities include the prompt and accurate setup of monitoring electrodes and systems, ensuring smooth data recording, and effectively troubleshooting any technical issues that may arise. The core of the intraoperative function is maintaining high attentiveness in the analysis and interpretation of complex electrophysiological data (Bianchi and Del Carro 2024; Guzzi et al. 2024). The nurse must be adept at identifying subtle signal changes that could indicate potential neurological compromise.

Immediate and clear communication is paramount. The nurse specialist provides real-time feedback to the surgical and anesthetic teams, alerting them to any significant changes in motor or sensory function. This collaborative loop is vital for preventing permanent neurological damage (Bianchi and Del Carro 2024; Guzzi et al. 2024; Oliva et al. 2023). This includes working with anesthesiologists to optimize an anesthetic regimen, as certain agents can interfere with electrophysiological signals. Throughout the procedure, the nurse specialist upholds the highest standards of patient safety, adhering to strict infection control protocols for needle electrode insertion and equipment policies for electrical stimulation (Guzzi et al. 2024; Oliva et al. 2023).

Postoperative Phase: Continuity of Care and Rehabilitation

The nurse specialist's involvement extends into the postoperative phase to ensure a seamless continuity of care. They perform follow-up assessments to monitor the patient's progress and evaluate their neurological status. This evaluation is instrumental in the early identification of any functional deficits. By integrating IONM findings with overall patient assessments, the nurse specialist plays a pivotal role in initiating a postoperative rehabilitation plan (Shady et al. 2025). This involves collaborating with a multidisciplinary team to arrange for necessary therapies, develop coping strategies for any new neurological deficits, and provide essential social and psychological support (Shady et al. 2025; Wang et al. 2024).

Advantages and Evaluation of the Nurse-Led Model

The nurse-led IONM service offers distinct advantages that enhance the quality and safety of patient care. Its patient-centered approach ensures that the patient's needs and emotional state are considered, providing a more integrated and holistic care dynamic (Shady et al. 2025). From a clinical standpoint, evidence-based practice has demonstrated significant benefits, including more complete resections for brain tumor cases with fewer permanent deficits, improved neurological outcomes for patients undergoing spinal tumor excision, and decreased rates of complications and unplanned readmissions (Bu et al. 2021; Gerritsen et al. 2019; Niljianskul and Prasertchai 2023; Ament et al. 2023).

The value of this service is recognized by both clinicians and patients. Neurosurgeons appreciate successful and reliable monitoring, effective communication and collaboration during procedures, and patient-centered focus. Patients reflect positive surgical outcomes due to effective IONM, a high quality of care marked by continuous monitoring, and benefit from clear explanations and dedicated patient advocacy.

The Nurse-Led Transcranial Doppler Service in Neurosurgical Care

Transcranial Doppler (TCD) is a noninvasive ultrasound method used to measure the velocity and direction of blood flow within the major intracranial arteries (Loomis and Chakko 2023; Sharma et al. 2019). Its principal application is in the assessment and ongoing management of patients with cerebrovascular diseases. Established clinical indications for TCD include the evaluation of sickle cell disease, cerebral ischemia, the detection of right-to-left shunts (RLS), monitoring during surgical procedures, and confirming brain death (Alexandrov et al. 2012; Ali 2021; Loomis and Chakko 2023). A particularly critical use is in the surveillance of patients following an aneurysmal subarachnoid hemorrhage (SAH) (Park et al. 2022).

Application for Vasospasm Monitoring

In the neurosurgical high-dependency setting, TCD is a cornerstone for monitoring patients who have suffered an aneurysmal SAH (Loomis and Chakko 2023; Park et al. 2022). The primary goal is to track blood flow velocities in the middle cerebral artery (MCA), posterior cerebral artery (PCA), and the intracranial portion of the internal carotid artery (ICA) (Jarrett et al. 2020; Park et al. 2022). This surveillance allows for the early detection of intracranial vasospasm, a dangerous narrowing of the cerebral arteries (Jarrett et al. 2020). Prompt identification and treatment of vasospasm are vital to prevent delayed cerebral ischemia, a complication that significantly contributes to the high rates of morbidity and mortality among SAH patients (Loomis and Chakko 2023; Park et al. 2022).

Key Hemodynamic Parameters and Interpretation

To quantify and interpret blood flow dynamics, specific parameters are investigated (Loomis and Chakko 2023):

- *Mean Cerebral Blood Flow Velocity (MFV)*: This value reflects the average velocity of blood flow over a cardiac cycle. It is calculated from the peak systolic velocity (PSV) and the end-diastolic velocity (EDV) using the formula: MFV = [PSV + (EDV × 2)]/3.
- *Lindegaard Ratio (LR)*: The LR is a critical calculated value that helps differentiate true vasospasm from hyperemia (a general increase in the blood flow), which can also present with elevated velocities (Puppo 2022). It is derived by dividing the MFV of the middle cerebral artery by the MFV of the ipsilateral internal carotid artery (Schenck et al. 2025). An elevated MCA velocity that is proportionally much higher than the ICA velocity points toward vasospasm as the cause (Park et al. 2022). The severity of vasospasm is graded based on this ratio (Park et al. 2022).
  The following values are commonly used to classify the degree of vasospasm in specific arteries (Loomis and Chakko 2023):
- *Middle Cerebral Artery (MCA)*:
  - *Normal*: MFV <120 cm/s and Lindegaard ratio <3.
  - *Mild Vasospasm*: MFV of 120–150 cm/s with a Lindegaard ratio of 3.0–4.5.
  - *Moderate Vasospasm*: MFV of 150–200 cm/s with a Lindegaard ratio of 4.5–6.0.
  - *Severe Vasospasm*: MFV >200 cm/s and a Lindegaard ratio >6.0.
- *Anterior Cerebral Artery (ACA)*: Vasospasm is indicated by an MFV greater than 80 cm/s.
- *Posterior Cerebral Artery (PCA)*: Vasospasm is indicated by an MFV greater than 85 cm/s.

The Enhanced Role of the Nurse-Led Service

The integration of TCD monitoring into the responsibilities of a nurse specialist team represents a significant advancement in patient care. In this model, nurses perform daily TCD surveillance, often for the first 2 weeks following a ruptured aneurysm, a critical period for vasospasm development (Samagh et al. 2019). The advantage of a nurse-led service extends beyond the technical performance and reporting of TCD findings (Wang et al. 2024). Nurse specialists are uniquely positioned to synthesize the sonographic data with their continuous assessment of the patient's neurological status and overall clinical progress. This holistic understanding facilitates more effective and timely communication with the neurological team, ensuring that TCD results are interpreted within the full clinical context (Park et al. 2022; Wang et al. 2024). This integrated approach is crucial for optimizing clinical management decisions and ultimately enhancing patient outcomes.

Conclusion

In Hong Kong, the integration of a neurosurgical nurse specialist team establishes a comprehensive, patient-centered model of care, prioritizing early rapport-building to understand patient and family concerns. Through advanced nurse-led services, including specialized clinics, intraoperative monitoring, and case management, this team significantly enhances patient safety and optimizes surgical outcomes. This holistic approach ensures a seamless continuum of care across all surgical phases, facilitating a smooth transition from hospital to home or other facilities and fostering multidisciplinary collaboration for superior clinical results within Hong Kong's demanding healthcare environment.

References

Alexandrov AV, Sloan MA, Tegeler CH, Newell DN, Lumsden A, Garami Z, Levy CR, Wong LKS, Douville C, Kaps M, Tsivgoulis G, American Society of Neuroimaging Practice Guidelines Committee (2012) Practice standards for transcranial Doppler (TCD) ultrasound. Part II Clinical indications and expected outcomes. J Neuroimaging 22(3):215–224. https://doi.org/10.1111/j.1552-6569.2010.00523.x

Ali MF (2021) Transcranial doppler ultrasonography (uses, limitations, and potentials): a review article. Egypt J Neurosurg 36(20):1–9. https://doi.org/10.1186/s41984-021-00114-0

Alvarez CM, Farhan R, Jahangiri FR (2023) Benefits of intraoperative neurophysiological monitoring (IONM) for the localization, mapping, and resection of tumors in the fourth ventricle: a literature review. J Neurophysiol Monit 1(1):22–36. https://doi.org/10.5281/zenodo.10207910

Ament JD, Leon A, Kim KD, Johnson JP, Vokshoor A (2023) Intraoperative neuromonitoring in spine surgery: large database analysis of cost-effectiveness. N Am Spine Soc J 14:100206. https://doi.org/10.1016/j.xnsj.2023.100206

Bianchi F, Del Carro U (2024) Intraoperative neurophysiological monitoring in neurosurgery. In: Neurosurgical treatment of central nervous system tumors. Springer, Cham, pp 33–48. https://doi.org/10.1007/978-3-031-68578-1_3

Bu LH, Zhang J, Lu JF, Wu JS (2021) Glioma surgery with awake language mapping versus generalized anesthesia: a systematic review. Neurosurg Rev 44(4):1997–2011. https://doi.org/10.1007/s10143-020-01418-9

Cartwright C, Kennedy L (2025) A blueprint for the future: why the "call to action" in acute and critical care nursing matters to neuroscience nursing. J Neurosci Nurs 57:150–151. https://doi.org/10.1097/JNN.0000000000000836

Errico M, Luoma AMV (2023) Postoperative care of neurosurgical patients: general principles. Anaesth Intensive Care Med 24(5):282–290. https://doi.org/10.1016/j.mpaic.2023.03.011

Gerritsen JKW, Arends L, Klimek M, Dirven CMF, Vincent AJPE (2019) Impact of intraoperative stimulation mapping on high-grade glioma surgery outcome: a meta-analysis. Acta Neurochir 161(1):99–107. https://doi.org/10.1007/s00701-018-3732-4

Goonasekera C, Smith EJ (eds) (2021) The basics of intra-operative neurophysiological monitoring for the clinician: a practical guide. Cambridge Scholars Publishing

Guldager R, Loft MI, Nordentoft S, Aadal L, Poulsen I (2022) Facilitators and barriers of relatives' involvement in nursing care decisions and self-care of patients with acquired brain injury or malignant brain tumour: a scoping review protocol. PLoS One 17(8):e0273151. https://doi.org/10.1371/journal.pone.0273151

Guzzi G, Ricciuti RA, Della Torre A, Lo Turco E, Lavano A, Longhini F, La Torre D (2024) Intraoperative neurophysiological monitoring in neurosurgery. J Clin Med 13(10):2966. https://doi.org/10.3390/jcm13102966

Hospital Authority, Strategy and Planning Division (2016) Clinical services plan for the Kowloon central cluster. Hospital Authority. Retrieved from https://www.ha.org.hk/haho/ho/ap/CSP-KCC_2.pdf

Ibrahim NM, Qalawa SAA, Mohamed NA, Ibrahim AM (2025) An in-depth analysis of nurses' knowledge, practice, and attitude towards neurological examination and the challenges: "bridging the gap". BMC Nurs 24(1):213. https://doi.org/10.1186/s12912-025-02766-x

Institute of Advanced Nursing Studies (2024) Post-registration certification course in neuroscience nursing 2024/25. Hospital Authority. Retrieved from https://www26.ha.org.hk/CourseOutline/G4896_00001_001.pdf

Jarrett CL, Shields KL, Broxterman RM, Hydren JR, Park SH, Gifford JR, Richardson RS (2020) Imaging transcranial Doppler ultrasound to measure middle cerebral artery blood flow: the importance of measuring vessel diameter. Am J Phys Regul Integr Comp Phys 319(1):R33–R42. https://doi.org/10.1152/ajpregu.00025.2020

Kumar GK, Pradeep K, Rajesh BJ, Bhaire VS, Manohar N, Balasubramaniam A (2021) Intraoperative electrophysiological principles in neurooncological practice. Int J Neurooncol 4(Suppl 1):S147–S163. https://doi.org/10.4103/IJNO.IJNO_421_21

Lee KS, Yordanov S, Stubbs D, Edlmann E, Joannides A, Davies B (2021) Integrated care pathways in neurosurgery: a systematic review. PLoS One 16(8):e0255628. https://doi.org/10.1371/journal.pone.0255628

Lindlöf J, Turunen H, Coco K, Huhtakangas J, Verhaeghe S, Välimäki T (2024) Empowering support for family members of patients with traumatic brain injury during the acute care: insights from family members and nurses. J Adv Nurs 0:1–16. https://doi.org/10.1111/jan.16424

Loomis AL, Chakko MN (2023) Doppler trans-cranial assessment, protocols, and interpretation, National Institutes of Health. Retrieved from https://www.ncbi.nlm.nih.gov/books/NBK570636/

Miao Q, Yan Y, Zhou M, Sun X (2023) The role of nursing care in the management of patients with traumatic subarachnoid hemorrhage. Galen Med J 12:e3013. https://doi.org/10.31661/gmj.v12i.3013

Mofatteh M, Mashayekhi MS, Arfaie S, Adeleye AO, Jolayemi EO, Ghomsi NC, JShlobin NA, Morsy AA, Esene IN, Laeke T, Awad AK, Labuschagne JJ, Ruan R, Abebe YN, Jabang JN, Okunlola AI, Barrie U, Lekuya HM, Idi Marcel E, Kabulo KDM, Bankole NDA, Edem IJ, Kkwuegbuenyi CA, Nguembu S, Zolo Y, Bernstein M (2023) Awake craniotomy in Africa: a scoping review of literature and proposed solutions to tackle challenges. Neurosurgery 93(2):274–291. https://doi.org/10.1227/neu.0000000000002453

Niljianskul N, Prasertchai P (2023) The effect of intraoperative neurophysiological monitoring on neurological outcomes after spinal tumors operations: a single institution experience. Interdiscip Neurosurg 31:101703. https://doi.org/10.1016/j.inat.2022.101703

Oliva AM, Montejano J, Simmons CG, Vogel SA, Isaza CF, Clavijo CF (2023) New frontiers in intraoperative neurophysiologic monitoring: a narrative review. Ann Transl Med 11(11):388. https://doi.org/10.21037/atm-22-4586

Oteri V, Martinelli A, Crivellaro E, Gigli F (2021) The impact of preoperative anxiety on patients undergoing brain surgery: a systematic review. Neurosurg Rev 44(6):3047–3057. https://doi.org/10.1007/s10143-021-01498-1

Park SH, Kim TJ, Ko SB (2022) Transcranial doppler monitoring in subarachnoid hemorrhage. J Neurosonol Neuroimaging *14*(1):1–9. https://doi.org/10.31728/jnn.2022.00115

Pugh JD, McCoy K, Needham M, Jiang L, Giles M, McKinnon E, Heine K (2022) Evaluation of an Australian neurological nurse-led model of postdischarge care. Health Soc Care Community 30(4):e962–e973. https://doi.org/10.1111/hsc.13498

Puppo C (2022) Neurosonology in the ICU: transcranial doppler (TCD) protocol. In: Rodríguez CN et al (eds) Neurosonology in critical care. Springer, Cham. https://doi.org/10.1007/978-3-030-81419-9_12

Roland JL, Hacker CD, Leuthardt EC (2021) A review of passive brain mapping techniques in neurological surgery. Neurosurgery 88(1):15–24. https://doi.org/10.1093/neuros/nyaa361

Samagh N, Bhagat H, Jangra K (2019) Monitoring cerebral vasospasm: how much can we rely on transcranial doppler. J Anaesthesiol Clin Pharmacol 35(1):12–18. https://doi.org/10.4103/joacp.JOACP_192_17

Schenck H, van Craenenbroeck C, van Kuijk S, Gommer E, Veldeman M, Temel Y, Aries M, Mess W, Haeren R (2025) Systematic review and meta-analysis of transcranial doppler biomarkers for the prediction of delayed cerebral ischemia following subarachnoid hemorrhage. J Cereb Blood Flow Metab 45(6):1031–1047. https://doi.org/10.1177/0271678X251313746

Shady RHA, El-Shaboury RHR, Elsaid RAA, Ahmed SAEM, Badawy GG, Hamed WE, El-Etreby RR, Senosy AMK (2025) Enhancing nursing practice through patient outcome measures: a framework for optimizing care in intracranial surgery. BMC Nurs 24(1):402. https://doi.org/10.1186/s12912-025-02960-x

Sharma S, Lubrica RJ, Song M, Vandse R, Boling W, Pillai P (2019) The role of transcranial Doppler in cerebral vasospasm: a literature review. Subarachnoid Hemorrhage Neurol Care Protect 127:201–205. https://doi.org/10.1007/978-3-030-04615-6_32

Wang J, Wu Z, Shi S, Ren J, Ren X (2024) Nurse-led care versus neurologist-led care for long-term outcomes of patients who underwent craniotomy in traumatic brain injuries: an efficacy analysis. Front Neurol 15:1382696. https://doi.org/10.3389/fneur.2024.1382696

Wilson JP Jr, Vallejo JB, Kumbhare D, Guthikonda B, Hoang S (2023) The use of intraoperative neuromonitoring for cervical spine surgery: indications, challenges, and advances. J Clin Med 12(14):4652. https://doi.org/10.3390/jcm12144652

Yip A, Yip J, Tsui Z, Yip CH, Lung HL, Shit KY, Yip R (2025) The impact of COVID on healthcare services, risk management, and infection prevention in surgical settings: a qualitative study. Healthcare 13:579. https://doi.org/10.3390/healthcare13060579

Zentner J, MacDonald DB, Wegner C (eds) (2024) Intraoperative neuromonitoring: fundamentals, possibilities, limitations. Springer

Embracing the Future of Theatre Nursing: Hybrid Operating Rooms and Quality Assurance in Pathology

Cheung-Hai Yip and Alice Yip

Introduction

The adoption of hybrid operating rooms (ORs) is increasing in hospitals globally (Patel et al. 2020). The increasing prevalence of minimally invasive and endoscopic procedures will necessitate a corresponding rise in the demand of hybrid ORs (Casar Berazaluce et al. 2019; Chan et al. 2020). The hybrid OR represents an innovative advancement in preoperative nursing, integrating advanced imaging modalities with a multifunctional surgical table (Figs. 3.1 and 3.2) (Deng et al. 2023). This integrated approach facilitates both diagnostic and therapeutic procedures within a single setting, reducing risks associated with procedural delays and patient transfers. The field of surgery has experienced substantial advancements in recent years, notably driven by innovations in imaging technology, which have facilitated the development and adoption of minimally invasive surgical techniques (Ilcheva et al. 2023; Peters et al. 2018). These minimally invasive techniques offer numerous advantages, including diminished postoperative pain, increased recovery times, and a reduced incidence of postoperative complications. Patients undergoing hybrid procedures frequently exhibit a decreased length of hospital stay attributable to faster recovery and a lower incidence of postoperative complications such as bleeding and infection (Loftus et al. 2021; Low et al. 2019).

Numerous specimens are submitted to pathology departments daily. Any error in specimen identification can have profound consequences, particularly within the

C.-H. Yip (✉)
Department of Anesthesiology & Operating Suite, Alice Ho Miu Ling Nethersole Hospital, Tai Po, HKSAR, China
e-mail: ych670@ha.org.hk

A. Yip
School of Health Sciences, St. Francis University, Tseung Kwan O, Hong Kong
e-mail: khyip@sfu.edu.hk

A. Yip, G. D. Smith (eds.), *Surgical Nursing in Practice*,
https://doi.org/10.1007/978-3-032-14729-5_3

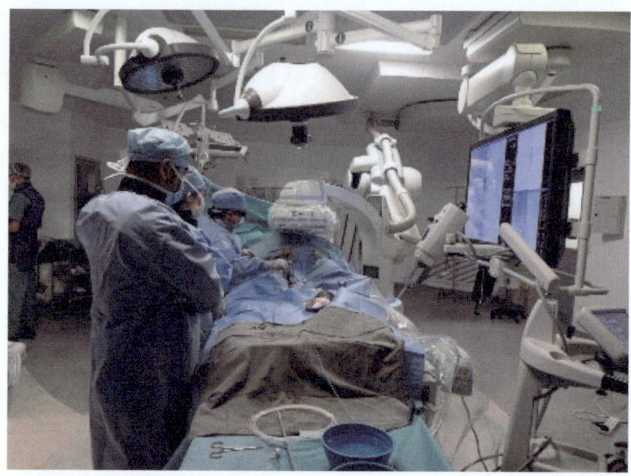

Fig. 3.1 Surgical procedure performed in hybrid OR

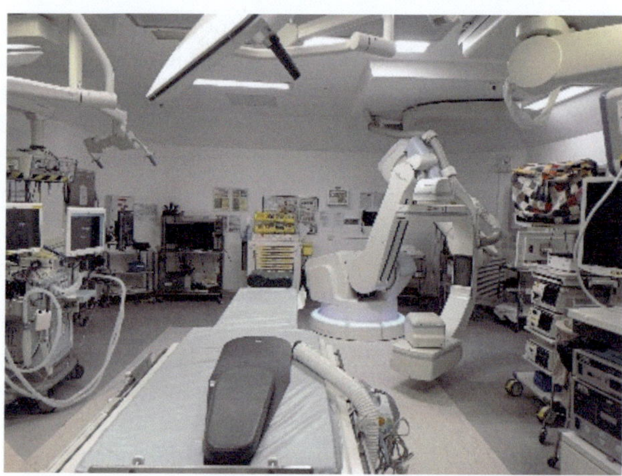

Fig. 3.2 A hybrid OR combines a surgical suite with advanced medical imaging capabilities

domain of diagnostic anatomical pathology (Fraggetta et al. 2021). The implementation of barcode technology has significantly enhanced sample tracking, mitigated errors, and improved overall workflow efficiency. Furthermore, radio frequency identification (RFID) demonstrates considerable potential for minimizing specimen loss and labelling errors throughout the pre-analytic and analytic phases of the pathology workflow (Profetto et al. 2022). However, further refinement of RFID technology is required prior to its widespread implementation within healthcare settings. The future of perioperative nursing hinges upon the continued development and integration of advanced technologies, such as hybrid ORs, and robust quality assurance measures within pathology services. These advancements will ultimately enhance patient care and improve treatment outcomes, especially for patients in surgical settings.

Hybrid OR

Hybrid ORs integrate advanced medical imaging modalities, such as fixed C-arms, X-ray computed tomography (CT) scanners, or magnetic resonance imaging (MRI) scanners, with a multifunctional surgical table (Esposito et al. 2020; Jin et al. 2022) (Figs. 3.3 and 3.4). This configuration enables surgeons and interdisciplinary teams to perform both diagnostic and therapeutic procedures within a single, integrated environment. The availability of real-time intraoperative imaging and computer-assisted instrument control facilitates enhanced precision and efficiency (Patel et al. 2020). Furthermore, the hybrid OR fosters multidisciplinary collaboration among specialists from various fields, enabling the execution of complex surgical procedures with enhanced speed, ease, safety, and minimally invasive techniques. These state-of-the-art facilities accommodate a wide spectrum of procedures, often less

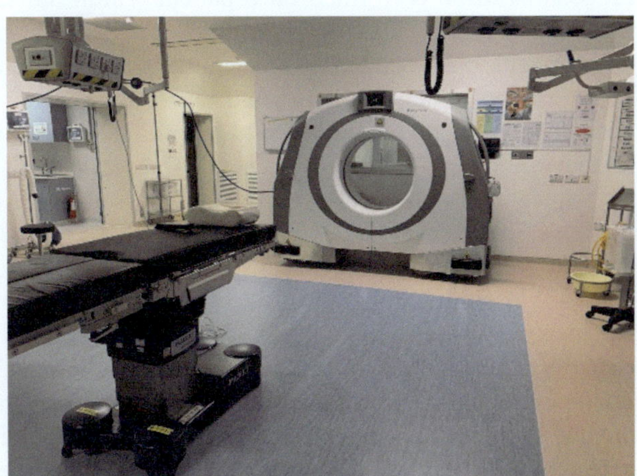

Fig. 3.3 Hybrid OR integrate advanced medical imaging modalities

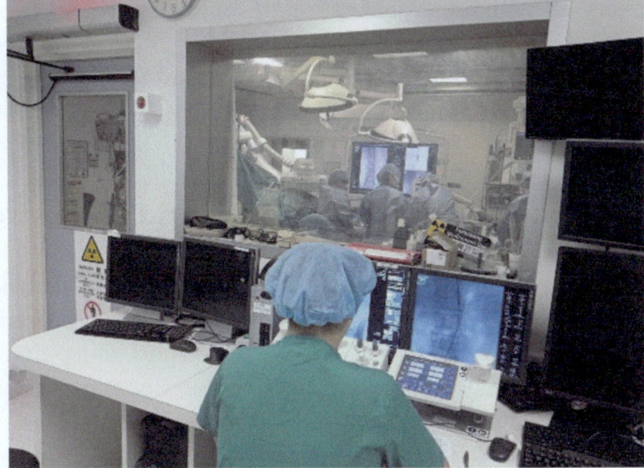

Fig. 3.4 Control room for hybrid OR: integration of advanced medical imaging modalities

invasive than traditional surgical approaches, resulting in expedited patient recovery (Jin et al. 2022; Patel et al. 2020). For instance, complex cardiovascular and endo-vascular conditions that previously necessitated open-heart surgery are now diag-nosed and treated using less invasive techniques within the hybrid OR environment (Esposito et al. 2020; Jin et al. 2022). The current primary applications of hybrid ORs include cardiac, vascular, neurosurgical, and orthopedic procedures.

Hybrid ORs: Advantages over Traditional Approaches

Recent decades have witnessed revolutionary advancements in surgical practice. The hybrid OR represents a significant innovation, integrating the functionalities of a traditional OR with advanced radiological imaging capabilities (Gharios et al. 2023). This integrated environment allows for both open surgical and interventional procedures to be performed on a patient within the same setting (Gharios et al. 2023; Zaffino et al. 2020). This inherent flexibility intraoperative conversion from an interventional procedure to an open surgical approach, if necessary (Zaffino et al. 2020; Zaman et al. 2024). Beyond representing a novel physical environment—characterized by increased space to accommodate personnel and advanced techno-logical equipment—the hybrid OR also necessitates a shift in team composition. This integrated approach offers patients less invasive diagnostic and therapeutic options (Gharios et al. 2023; Zaman et al. 2024).

Traditionally, patients with cardiovascular diseases, requiring procedures such as coronary artery bypass grafting, valve repair, or abdominal aortic aneurysm stent-ing, may necessitate examination and treatment across multiple hospital locations (Gharios et al. 2023). This often includes the radiology department for preoperative imaging and the catheterization laboratory for percutaneous interventions prior to the definitive surgical procedure. Postoperative reexploration occasionally become necessary after patients have been transferred to the intensive care unit. The hybrid OR, through the integration of diverse technologies, offers real-time, intraoperative imaging and computer-assisted instrument control. This empowers surgeons, physi-cians, and interventional radiologists to perform all necessary procedures within a single setting. Consequently, healthcare costs and hospital stays may be reduced, while treatment efficiency is enhanced and the risks associated with patient transfer are minimized (Gharios et al. 2023).

Nursing Practice Within the Hybrid OR Environment

From the perspective of nursing professionals, the demand for procedures amenable to the hybrid OR environment is increasing. Such procedures include thoracic endo-vascular aortic repair (TEVAR), single-port video-assisted thoracoscopic surgery (VATS) for major lung resection, and various image-guided surgical interventions (Fig. 3.5) (Gharios et al. 2023; Melloni et al. 2021). In the complex hybrid OR, nurses are pivotal in leading risk management and infection prevention to ensure patient safety, and their diverse skills and cohesive teamwork are crucial for navigating this

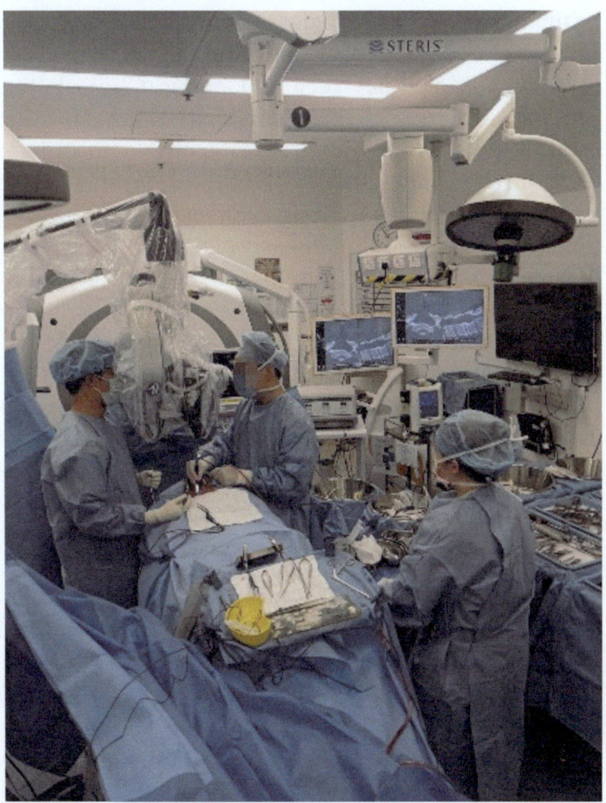

Fig. 3.5 Performing image-guided surgical interventions within a hybrid OR

high-tech environment, where advanced imaging and surgery merge (Yip et al. 2025). Furthermore, given the relative complexity of many procedures performed in the hybrid OR, nurses encounter numerous challenges, including OR setup, instrument preparation, and ensuring operative safety (Lang et al. 2024). A standardized template for basic OR setup and instrument preparation for various hybrid OR procedures is essential for nursing professionals to follow (Silverio et al. 2024). Methodical and organized placement of equipment and instruments is crucial. Furthermore, utilizing iPads as video teaching tools can provide nurses with increased opportunities for continuing education and access to updated knowledge. Mobile surgical instrument tracking system (SITS) facilitates instrument counting and issue reporting, offering an alternative communication method with sterile processing departments to ensure a smooth instrument workflow (van Nieuwenhuizen et al. 2024).

Specimen Tracking System Utilizing RFID

Specimen mishandling represents a preventable patient safety issue with the potential for serious adverse outcomes, particularly in the context of diagnostic anatomical pathology, where accurate specimen processing is essential for definitive disease diagnosis and subsequent treatment (Boulos and Attieh 2024). To mitigate patient risk associated with specimen handling errors and ensure appropriate treatment, quality control initiatives, including specimen tracking system utilizing technologies such as Generic Clinical Request System-Plus (GCRS-Plus), have been implemented in Hong Kong (Holstine and Samora 2021; Norgan et al. 2020). These systems verify physician orders and patient identification, often through integration with clinical dashboards, facilitating robust specimen tracking with the Hong Kong healthcare system. However, effective error mitigation necessitates a comprehensive approach addressing all stages of the specimen management process: from the pre-analytical phase encompassing sample collection, through the analytical phase within the laboratory, to the post-analytical phase, which includes diagnostic report delivery and archiving of pathological materials (Holstine and Samora 2021).

RFID technology offers a potential solution for enhancing the accuracy of specimen handling and mitigation the risk of errors (Norgan et al. 2020). By enabling continuous, automated tracking of specimens, RFID tags can minimize identification and tracking discrepancies, thereby improving the overall reliability of specimen management (Profetto et al. 2022). RFID is an automated wireless technology employing radio waves to facilitate remote data communication between an electronic tag and a reader. This technology is primarily utilized for identification and tracking purposes. Recent technological advancements have led to increased RFID adoption within hospital settings. RFID systems enable automated specimen tracking using small, wireless tags affixed to individual samples. The supporting scanning infrastructure is strategically deployed in laboratories and collection centers, facilitating real-time monitoring and management of the tagged specimens. Deploying RFID-based specimen tracking system (STS) can significantly mitigate the risk of specimen misidentification (Norgan et al. 2020). The process involves scanning the barcode on a patient's wristband to import patient demographics, typically performed by a nurse. Subsequently, an RFID tag printer generates a specimen tag containing both patient and specimen information. This automated procedure effectively reduces the potential for misidentification or transcription errors associated with illegible handwriting (Chen et al. 2022).

Upon placement of the tagged specimen container within the designated transporter and trolley, the embedded RFID tag enables automatic detection and reading the associated patient and specimen data. This information is then relayed to a specimen location tracking dashboard, providing real-time updates on the specimen's status and location (Chen et al. 2022). The utilization of RFID technology facilities automated detection and real-time traceability throughout the specimen handling process (Profetto et al. 2022). Furthermore, RFID-based STS incorporates a *found-missing* alert functionality (Chen et al. 2022). If a registered specimen is removed from the designated transporter or trolley and subsequently its location becomes unknown, an alert message is displayed on the tracking dashboard. This notification prompts nursing staff to investigate and clarify the specimen's status, thereby preventing inadvertent loss. Such robust specimen handling protocols contribute significantly to patient safety and mitigate potential adverse consequences (Chen et al. 2022).

Conclusion

This offers a strong concluding statement, the hybrid OR presents a novel paradigm of care. Advanced technologies within this setting may contribute to improved patient outcomes, facilitated by less invasive procedures, development and support of new surgical techniques, reduced lengths of hospital stay, fewer interventions and transfers, optimized resource utilization, and the acquisition of new skills, particularly for nursing professionals in both intraoperative and clinical ward settings. Interprofessional collaboration, unified by the common goal of delivering high-quality patient care, is essential. Furthermore, RFID specimen tracking not only mitigates potential specimen loss but also reduces the risk of misidentification or transcription errors associated with illegible handwriting. These advancements are crucial for the next generation of nursing professionals to understand and effectively implement updated practices within hybrid OR environments.

References

Boulos F, Attieh M (2024) Handling surgical specimens to decrease errors in pathology. In: Principles of perioperative safety and efficiency. Springer, Cham, pp 155–167. https://doi.org/10.1007/978-3-031-41089-5_10

Casar Berazaluce AM, Hanke RE, von Allmen D, Racadio JM (2019) The state of the hybrid operating room: technological acceleration at the pinnacle of collaboration. Curr Surg Rep 7:1–12. https://doi.org/10.1007/s40137-019-0229-x

Chan JW, Peter SY, Lau RW, Ng CS (2020) Hybrid operating room—one stop for diagnosis, staging and treatment of early stage NSCLC. J Thorac Dis 12(2):123. https://doi.org/10.21037/jtd.2019.08.36

Chen X, Yang K, Liu X, Xu Y, Luo J, Zhang S (2022) Efficient and accurate identification of missing tags for large-scale dynamic RFID systems. J Syst Archit 124:102394. https://doi.org/10.1016/j.sysarc.2022.102394

Deng Z, Xiang N, Pan J (2023) State of the art in immersive interactive technologies for surgery simulation: a review and prospective. Bioengineering 10(12):1346. https://doi.org/10.3390/bioengineering10121346

Esposito D, Gonfiantini F, Fargion AT, Dorigo W, Villani F, Di Domenico R, Speziali S, Pratesi C (2020) Hybrid operating room applications in the increasingly complex endovascular era: the trump card of modern vascular surgery. Ann Surg Treat Res 100(1):54. https://doi.org/10.4174/astr.2021.100.1.54

Fraggetta F, L'imperio V, Ameisen D, Carvalho R, Leh S, Kiehl TR, Serbanescu M, Racoceanu D, Della Mea V, Polonia A, Zerbe N, Eloy C (2021) Best practice recommendations for the implementation of a digital pathology workflow in the anatomic pathology laboratory by the European Society of Digital and Integrative Pathology (ESDIP). Diagnostics 11(11):2167. https://doi.org/10.3390/diagnostics11112167

Gharios M, El-Hajj VG, Frisk H, Ohlsson M, Omar A, Edström E, Elmi-Terander A (2023) The use of hybrid operating rooms in neurosurgery, advantages, disadvantages, and future perspectives: A systematic review. Acta Neurochir 165(9):2343–2358. https://doi.org/10.1007/s00701-023-05756-7

Holstine JB, Samora JB (2021) Reducing surgical specimen errors through multidisciplinary quality improvement. Jt Comm J Qual Patient Saf 47(9):563–571. https://doi.org/10.1016/j.jcjq.2021.04.003

Ilcheva L, Risteski P, Tudorache I, Häussler A, Papadopoulos N, Odavic D, Biefer HRC, Dzemali O (2023) Beyond conventional operations: embracing the era of contemporary minimally invasive cardiac surgery. J Clin Med 12(23):7210. https://doi.org/10.3390/jcm12237210

Jin H, Lu L, Liu J, Cui M (2022) A systematic review on the application of the hybrid operating room in surgery: experiences and challenges. Updat Surg:1–13. https://doi.org/10.1007/s13304-021-00989-6

Lang M, Duff J, Munday J (2024) Coordination of procedural equipment and supplies for the surgical set-up in the perioperative environment: A scoping review. J Perioper Nurs 37(4):e26–e38

Loftus TJ, Croft CA, Rosenthal MD, Mohr AM, Efron PA, Moore FA, Upchurch GR, Smith RS (2021) Clinical impact of a dedicated trauma hybrid operating room. J Am Coll Surg 232(4):560–570. https://doi.org/10.1016/j.jamcollsurg.2020.11.008

Low DE, Allum W, De Manzoni G, Ferri L, Immanuel A, Kuppusamy M, Law S, Lindblad M, Maynard N, Neal J, Pramesh CS, Scott M, Smithers BM, Addor V, Ljungqvist O (2019) Guidelines for perioperative care in esophagectomy: enhanced recovery after surgery (ERAS®) society recommendations. World J Surg 43:299–330. https://doi.org/10.1007/s00268-018-4786-4

Melloni G, Venturino M, Mazza F, Turello D (2021) Use of the hybrid room for thoracic surgery procedures: single-stage localization and removal of non-palpable nodules. Indian J Thorac Cardiovasc Surg 37(1):70–77. https://doi.org/10.1007/s12055-020-00997-y

Norgan AP, Simon KE, Feehan BA, Saari LL, Doppler JM, Welder GS, Sedarski J A, Yoch CT, Comfere NI, Martin JA, Bartholmai BJ, & Reichard RR (2020). Radio-frequency identification specimen tracking to improve quality in anatomic pathology. Archives of Pathology & Laboratory Medicine, 144(2), 189–195. https://doi.org/10.5858/arpa.2019-0011-OA

Patel S, Lindenberg M, Rovers MM, Van Harten WH, Ruers TJ, Poot L, Retel VP, Grutters JP (2020) Understanding the costs of surgery: a bottom-up cost analysis of both a hybrid operating room and conventional operating room. Int J Health Policy Manag 11(3):299. https://doi.org/10.34172/ijhpm.2020.119

Peters BS, Armijo PR, Krause C, Choudhury SA, Oleynikov D (2018) Review of emerging surgical robotic technology. Surg Endosc 32:1636–1655. https://doi.org/10.1007/s00464-018-6079-2

Profetto L, Gherardelli M, Iadanza E (2022) Radio frequency identification (RFID) in health care: where are we? A scoping review. Health Technol 12(5):879–891. https://doi.org/10.1007/s12553-022-00696-1

Silverio R, Al Nusair H, Latha P, Fonbuena M, Oidem N, Buenagua A, Sreenadh S (2024) Investigation of the perceptions of operating theatre nurses and central sterile supply department technicians regarding the barriers and facilitators of surgical instrument counts and tray management in the operating theatre. Perioper Care Oper Room Manag 35:100378. https://doi.org/10.1016/j.pcorm.2024.100378

van Nieuwenhuizen KE, van Trier T, Friedericy HJ, Jansen FW, Dankelman J, van der Eijk AC (2024) Optimising surgical instrument trays for sustainability and patient safety by combining actual instrument usage and expert recommendations. Sustainability 16(16):6953. https://doi.org/10.3390/su16166953

Yip A, Yip J, Tsui Z, Yip CH, Lung HL, Shit KY, Yip R (2025) The impact of COVID on healthcare services, risk management, and infection prevention in surgical settings: a qualitative study. Healthcare 13:579. https://doi.org/10.3390/healthcare13060579

Zaffino P, Moccia S, De Momi E, Spadea MF (2020) A review on advances in intra-operative imaging for surgery and therapy: imagining the operating room of the future. Ann Biomed Eng 48(8):2171–2191. https://doi.org/10.1007/s10439-020-02553-6

Zaman T, Williams AB, Singh T, Ellwood G, Williams Z (2024) The difficulties and solutions in operationalising a hybrid operating room. J Int Med Res 52(9):03000605241270700. https://doi.org/10.1177/03000605241270700

Enhancing Paediatric Surgical Care Through Team Collaboration and Advanced Enterostomal Therapy Skills

4

Zoe Tsui and Kam-Yee Shit

Introduction

Paediatric surgical nursing represents a specialized domain requiring advanced clinical expertise, profound understanding of child development, and a commitment to family-centred care (Hodgson et al. 2024). Children aged 0–18 years present unique physiological, emotional, and psychosocial challenges, compounded by the complex nature of surgical interventions (Gabriel et al. 2018). In Hong Kong, paediatric surgical nursing care has evolved to address the growing demand for specialized services tailored to the local population's needs. Nurses, as central figures in the care continuum, must possess advanced competencies in enterostomal therapy (ET) and leverage multidisciplinary team collaboration to optimize patient outcomes.

This chapter explores the integration of team collaboration and sophisticated ET nursing practices in paediatric surgical care. It highlights key programs that address critical areas, such as stoma management, complex wound care, anorectal and urological dysfunctions, and family education. By adopting evidence-based approaches and fostering a culture of trust and collaboration, paediatric nurses can significantly enhance the quality of care for Hong Kong's paediatric surgical population.

Z. Tsui (✉)
S.K. Yee School of Health Sciences, Saint Francis University,
Tseung Kwan O, HKSAR, China
e-mail: ztsui@sfu.edu.hk

K.-Y. Shit
Prince of Wales Hospital, Shatin, HKSAR, China
e-mail: sky366@ha.org.hk

Family-Centred Care and Advocacy

Children's mental well-being is significantly impacted by the considerable anxiety they often feel during surgical interventions or procedures. A child's emotional distress negatively impacts surgical recovery (Ma et al. 2025). In Hong Kong, family-centred care, which is integral to paediatric nursing, directly addresses this (Phiri et al. 2022; Tsui et al. 2023). Rooted in cultural values that emphasize the family's central role in healthcare decisions, this approach involves families in their child's care. This collaboration reduces anxiety, leading to better surgical outcomes. ET nurses adopt a culturally competent approach, addressing the diverse beliefs and practices that influence family dynamics and caregiving roles (Aubel et al. 2021; Zhang et al. 2021).

Advanced counselling skills are employed to support families in navigating the challenges of paediatric surgical care (Ma et al. 2025; Ratta et al. 2025). This includes providing clear and empathetic explanations of complex medical information, addressing emotional concerns, and connecting families with community resources (Hodgson et al. 2024). The empowerment of families as collaborative partners in the paediatric surgical process is achieved by ET nurses through strategic interventions; these include establishing clear lines of communication to build trust, alongside providing psychoeducational support, which collectively foster a safer and more supportive care environment (Ma et al. 2025).

Advanced Paediatric Stoma Care Education

The care of paediatric patients with stomas, such as colostomies, ileostomies, or urostomies, requires highly specialized nursing skills (Panattoni et al. 2023). In Hong Kong, the Paediatric Stoma Care Program integrates advanced ET practices to address the unique anatomical and developmental variations in children (Specialty Advisory Group (Enterostomal Therapy) 2025). Preoperative preparation includes detailed anatomical assessment, psychological readiness evaluations, and individualized stoma site marking, ensuring optimal placement that considers growth, mobility, and lifestyle.

Post-operatively, ET nurses play a crucial role in managing complications such as mucocutaneous separation, stoma prolapse, and peristomal skin issues (Specialty Advisory Group (Enterostomal Therapy) 2025). Techniques such as pressure-release dressing, advanced skin barrier products, and nascent technologies like silicone-based wound adhesives are utilized. They provide culturally sensitive guidance that addresses the intersection of emotional distress, such as fear and anxiety, with the practical challenges of dietary adjustments for stoma care, a vital role within cultural contexts that emphasize traditional dietary norms (Ma et al. 2025). Regular follow-ups ensure that stoma care evolves with the child's growth and developmental milestones.

Management of Complex Paediatric Wounds

Paediatric surgical wounds, often complicated by comorbidities, require advanced wound care strategies tailored to the child's unique physiological healing processes (McNamara et al. 2020). ET nurses employ cutting-edge techniques, such as anti-microbial hydrocolloids, and bioengineered skin substitutes, like allografts and xenografts.

A comprehensive assessment plan is employed, which includes evaluating infection risks, psychosocial factors, and nutritional status. Pain management during dressing changes is a priority, with interventions such as procedural sedation, child-directed distraction tools, and cognitive-behavioural therapy (CBT) integrated into care (Friedrichsdorf and Goubert 2020; McNamara et al. 2020). ET nurses collaborate with dietitians and physiotherapists to optimize wound healing through nutritional supplementation and mobility programs, respectively (Alsuroor et al. 2024).

Comprehensive Paediatric Bowel Management

The paediatric anorectal manometry and biofeedback plan addresses the management of functional bowel disorders, such as faecal incontinence, and chronic constipation in children with conditions like Hirschsprung's disease or anorectal malformations (Yates et al. 2021). By employing high-resolution manometry systems, specially trained ET nurses can conduct in-depth evaluations of anorectal physiology. Their assessment of functions like recto-anal coordination, reflexes, and rectal sensation provides the necessary insights to design effective, individualized care plans for patients (Athanasakos and Cleeve 2022; Scott and Carrington 2020).

Biofeedback therapy for paediatric faecal incontinence is a rehabilitative approach that targets the neuromuscular mechanisms of bowel control (Afonso et al. 2024; Yates et al. 2021). Delivered through interactive platforms designed for children, it provides real-time auditory or visual feedback on pelvic feedback on pelvic floor muscle activity and anorectal pressure. This process aims to enhance pelvic floor muscle coordination and improve rectal sensory awareness, which are often impaired in children with this condition (Afonso et al. 2024). Nurses are central to managing paediatric conditions like faecal incontinence, functional constipation, pelvic floor dyssynergia, and anorectal pain. They provide crucial counselling to families, guiding them on dietary adjustments, structured toileting regimes, and emotional coping strategies while emphasizing the importance of adhering to the overall treatment plan. The integration of culturally tailored educational resources ensures that families are well-equipped to support their child's progress.

The paediatric bowel management plan is a multidisciplinary initiative aimed at achieving continence and improving the quality of life for children with functional constipation (Vriesman et al. 2020). ET nurses are skilled in formulating individualized bowel management programs. They strategically combine pharmacological treatments, such as stimulant laxatives and osmotic agents, with mechanical therapies like enemas or transanal irrigation to create a comprehensive care plan.

In the Hong Kong context, dietary counselling often incorporates traditional Chinese medicine (TCM) principles alongside Western approaches, recognizing the cultural significance of certain foods and herbs (Wei et al. 2023). Nurses provide ongoing monitoring and adjust management plans in response to the child's growth and developmental changes. Psychosocial support is also integral, with nurses addressing the stigma often associated with bowel dysfunction and promoting self-esteem in affected children (Paknejad et al. 2019; Tan et al. 2025).

Urodynamic Studies in Paediatric Nursing

Urodynamic studies are essential for diagnosing and managing paediatric urinary tract dysfunctions, such as neurogenic bladder and vesicoureteral reflux (Hobbs et al. 2021; Kopač 2024). ET nurses are adept at conducting these studies, utilizing advanced technologies like video urodynamics and electromyography (EMG) to assess bladder and urethral function during voiding.

A child-centred approach is crucial in this domain. Nurses use age-appropriate educational tools, such as videos and anatomical models, to prepare children for the procedure (Kopač 2024). Collaboration with urologists, physiotherapists, and psychologists ensures comprehensive care, addressing both the physiological and emotional aspects of urinary dysfunction.

Paediatric Clean Intermittent Catheterization (CIC) Program

The Paediatric Clean Intermittent Catheterization Program equips children and their families with the knowledge and skills to perform safe and effective catheterization (Bauer et al. 2023a, b). ET nurses provide hands-on training sessions, using simulation models to build confidence and minimize procedural anxiety.

In Hong Kong, the program emphasizes infection prevention through the use of closed-system catheters and stringent hygiene practices. Nurses also address the psychosocial impact of catheterization, particularly in adolescents, by advocating for school-based support systems and peer education programs to reduce stigma (Hayes et al. 2022).

Urotherapy and Biofeedback in Paediatric Care

The Paediatric Urotherapy and Biofeedback Program combines advanced nursing interventions with innovative technologies to manage urinary incontinence and voiding dysfunctions (Wijekoon and Deshpande 2024). ET nurses deliver individualized therapy sessions that include bladder training, pelvic floor muscle exercises, and biofeedback using child-friendly interfaces.

A critical component of this program is family engagement. Nurses provide detailed explanations of treatment goals and encourage parents to actively participate in therapy sessions. The use of culturally relevant educational materials, such as bilingual guides and videos, ensures that families from diverse backgrounds are well-informed and supported.

Multidisciplinary Team Collaboration

In Hong Kong, multidisciplinary team collaboration is a cornerstone of paediatric surgical care. Regular multidisciplinary meetings, shared care plans, and joint clinics facilitate seamless communication and coordination among surgeons, ET nurses, psychologists, dietitians, and social workers. ET nurses advocate for paediatric patients and their families by ensuring care plans are tailored to their unique needs and by taking a leadership role in fostering a team culture of mutual respect and shared decision-making, which is essential for delivering holistic, patient-centred care.

Conclusion

Paediatric surgical nursing in Hong Kong demands a high level of clinical expertise, cultural competence, and commitment to multidisciplinary collaboration. By integrating advanced enterostomal therapy skills with a family-centred approach, nurses can address the unique challenges of paediatric surgical care and improve outcomes for children and their families.

This chapter has highlighted the critical role of paediatric nurses in programs, such as stoma care, wound management, and bowel and urological therapy, emphasizing the importance of evidence-based practices and culturally tailored interventions. As the field continues to evolve, ongoing professional development, research, and innovation will be essential in ensuring that Hong Kong's paediatric population receives the highest standard of surgical nursing care.

References

Afonso SC, Ramalhao NC, Cavalheiro A, Trepa A (2024) Biofeedback therapy in managing functional fecal incontinence in children: a literature review. Cureus 16(11). https://doi.org/10.7759/cureus.74295

Alsuroor NFN, Alrshidi FS, Alzaid MNF, Awaji TMM, Faqihi AHA, Alotaibi AS, Al-Tamimi, Raghian S, Aldawood ASS (2024) Optimizing postoperative recovery: the synergy between physiotherapy, nursing, nutrition, and pharmacy. J Int Crisis Risk Commun Res 7(S11):1489. https://doi.org/10.63278/jicrcr.vi.1417

Athanasakos E, Cleeve S (2022) Anorectal manometry, conventional and high resolution in paediatrics. In: Lima M, Ruggeri G (eds) Ano-rectal endosonography and manometry in paediatrics. Springer, Cham. https://doi.org/10.1007/978-3-030-97668-2_6

Aubel J, Martin SL, Cunningham K (2021) Introduction: a family systems approach to promote maternal, child and adolescent nutrition. Matern Child Nutr 17:e13228. https://doi.org/10.1111/mcn.13228

Bauer SB, Choung K, Sable P, Dykeman BS, Venna A, Shanahan M, Sexton KE, Price DE, Hayes LC, Tham RL, Christensen S, Sullivan K (2023a) The impact of clean intermittent catheterization on students and families in the school environment. Neurourol Urodyn 42(8):1702–1711. https://doi.org/10.1002/nau.25271

Bauer SB, Saunders RA, Masoom SN, Choung K, Hayes LC, Price DE, Keays M, Sable PE, Shimmel A (2023b) The art of introducing clean intermittent catheterization: how families respond and adapt: a qualitative study. Neurourol Urodyn 42(1):309–321. https://doi.org/10.1002/nau.25085

Friedrichsdorf SJ, Goubert L (2020) Pediatric pain treatment and prevention for hospitalized children. Pain Rep 5(1):e804. https://doi.org/10.1097/PR9.0000000000000804

Gabriel MG, Wakefield CE, Vetsch J, Karpelowsky JS, Darlington ASE, Grant DM, Signorelli C (2018) The psychosocial experiences and needs of children undergoing surgery and their parents: a systematic review. J Pediatr Health Care 32(2):133–149. https://doi.org/10.1016/j.pedhc.2017.08.003

Hayes LC, Meers A, Tulley K, Sable PE, Castagno S, Cilento BG (2022) Interdisciplinary collaboration in a pediatric urology outpatient clinic at a tertiary children's hospital: a case series. Urology 169:191–195. https://doi.org/10.1016/j.urology.2022.07.036

Hobbs KT, Krischak M, Tejwani R, Purves JT, Wiener JS, Routh JC (2021) The importance of early diagnosis and management of pediatric neurogenic bladder dysfunction. Res Rep Urol:647–657. https://doi.org/10.2147/RRU.S259307

Hodgson CR, Mehra R, Franck LS (2024) Child and family outcomes and experiences related to family-centered care interventions for hospitalized pediatric patients: a systematic review. Children 11(8):949. https://doi.org/10.3390/children11080949

Kopač M (2024) Pediatric lower urinary tract dysfunction: a comprehensive exploration of clinical implications and diagnostic strategies. Biomedicine 12(5):945. https://doi.org/10.3390/biomedicines12050945

Ma X, Zhang Z, Bao Y, Zhao H (2025) Impact of pediatric surgery on anxiety in children and their families and coping strategies: a narrative review. Translat Pediatr 14(4):718. https://doi.org/10.21037/tp-2025-10

McNamara SA, Hirt PA, Weigelt MA, Nanda S, de Bedout V, Kirsner RS, Schachner LA (2020) Traditional and advanced therapeutic modalities for wounds in the paediatric population: an evidence-based review. J Wound Care 29(6):321–334. https://doi.org/10.12968/jowc.2020.29.6.321

Paknejad MS, Motaharifard MS, Barimani S, Kabiri P, Karimi M (2019) Traditional, complementary and alternative medicine in children constipation: A systematic review. DARU J Pharma Sci 27(2):811–826. https://doi.org/10.1007/s40199-019-00297-w

Panattoni N, Mariani R, Spano A, Leo AD, Iacorossi L, Petrone F, Simone ED (2023) Nurse specialist and ostomy patient: competence and skills in the care pathway. A scoping review. J Clin Nurs 32(17–18):5959–5973. https://doi.org/10.1111/jocn.16722

Phiri PG, Chan CW, Wong CL, Choi KC, Ng MS (2022) Discrepancies between nurses' current and perceived necessary practices of family-centred care for hospitalised children and their families: a cross-sectional study. J Pediatr Nurs 62:e25–e31. https://doi.org/10.1016/j.pedn.2021.06.021

Ratta BS, Kekre G, Vaze D, Kulkarni K (2025) Surgical decision-making in difficult situations in pediatric surgery. In: Surgical decision-making: evidence and beyond. Springer Nature Switzerland, Cham, pp 159–170. https://doi.org/10.1007/978-3-031-67391-7_14

Scott SM, Carrington EV (2020) The London classification: improving characterization and classification of anorectal function with anorectal manometry. Curr Gastroenterol Rep 22(11):55

Specialty Advisory Group (Enterostomal Therapy) (2025) Patient education series: paediatric stoma care. Hospital Authority. Online available: https://www.smartpatient.ha.org.hk/docs/default-source/disease-pdf/paediatric-stoma-care.pdf?sfvrsn=d11364bf_4. Accessed on 3 Sept 2025

Tan S, Peng C, Lin X, Peng C, Yang Y, Liu S, Huang L, Bian Y, Li Y, Xu C (2025) Clinical efficacy of non-pharmacological treatment of functional constipation: a systematic review and network meta-analysis. Front Cell Infect Microbiol 15:1565801. https://doi.org/10.3389/fcimb.2025.1565801

Tsui WK, Yip KH, Yip YC (2023) Heartbreak and loneliness due to family separations and limited visiting during COVID-19: a qualitative study. Int J Environ Res Public Health 20(2):1633. https://doi.org/10.3390/ijerph20021633

Vriesman MH, Koppen IJN, Camilleri M, Di Lorenzo C, Benninga MA (2020) Management of functional constipation in children and adults. Nat Rev Gastroenterol Hepatol 17:21–39. https://doi.org/10.1038/s41575-019-0222-y

Wei DJ, Li HJ, Lyu ZP, Lyu AP, Bian ZX, Zhong LL (2023) A clinical pathway for integrative medicine in the treatment of functional constipation in Hong Kong, China. J Integr Med 21(6):550–560. https://doi.org/10.1016/j.joim.2023.11.002

Wijekoon N, Deshpande A (2024) Treatment modalities for paediatric functional daytime lower urinary tract disorders: an updated review. Ther Adv Urol 16:17562872241241848. https://doi.org/10.1177/17562872241241848

Yates G, Friedmacher F, Cleeve S, Athanasakos E (2021) Anorectal manometry in pediatric settings: a systematic review of 227 studies. Neurogastroenterol Motil 33(4):e14006. https://doi.org/10.1111/nmo.14006

Zhang X, Lin JL, Gao R, Chen N, Huang GF, Wang L, Gao H, Zhuo HZ, Chen LQ, Chen XH, Li H (2021) Application of the hospital-family holistic care model in caregivers of patients with permanent enterostomy: a randomized controlled trial. J Adv Nurs 77(4):2033–2049. https://doi.org/10.1111/jan.14691

Part II

Capability and Self-Care

Research and Education in Surgical Nursing

5

Graeme Drummond Smith

Introduction

Around the world, research and education constitute vital elements of contemporary surgical nursing. Representing one of the most critical nursing specialties, in which the provision of person-centered care is the cornerstone of high-quality care, surgical nursing requires important contributions from both research and education. Drawing upon evidence from surgical nursing practice and literature, local and international, this chapter aims to provide a comprehensive and relevant overview on the importance of research and education within the surgical nursing specialty.

Education in Surgical Nursing

Education plays an important role in the pathway of surgical nurses in Hong Kong. Evidence suggests that continued professional nurse education can significantly reduce the risk of errors in clinical environment and can increase patient confidence in surgical nurses (Audet et al. 2018). Through all aspects of surgical nursing from preoperative assessment through intraoperative and post-operative nursing care, education plays a vital role to support continuing professional development, ensuring that surgical nurses on the clinical frontline can remain updated in their clinical practice in relation to aspect of patient safety, infection control, and pain management (Vasilopoulos 2024). In recent years, technological advances have changed the global healthcare landscape, and the development and integration of patient monitoring systems and digital data collection systems have had a positive impact on surgical patient care. However, it is only through continuing education that surgical

G. D. Smith (✉)
School of Health Sciences, St. Francis University,
Tseung Kwan O, Hong Kong
e-mail: gsmith@sfu.edu.hk

   41
A. Yip, G. D. Smith (eds.), *Surgical Nursing in Practice*,
https://doi.org/10.1007/978-3-032-14729-5_5

nurses can attain the appropriate skill set that is required to ensure the delivery of safe and effective care using these technological innovations. Continuing professional education is essential to help develop competencies associated with all aspects of surgical nursing, like simulated based education. As such, ongoing continuing professional education helps to ensure that surgical nurses have the most up-to-date competencies for the delivery of optimal surgical nursing care. Therefore, within surgical nursing, education can offer numerous benefits that can improve both personal and professional development.

Education and the Surgical Career Pathways

The surgical nursing career pathway in Hong Kong is generally well-established, structured, and progressive, from foundational nursing education and practice leading to studying for higher degree and employment opportunities in more advanced clinical roles. Career development in surgical nursing may also ultimately lead to leadership opportunities and contribution to roles in nursing education and research. In general, the typical pathway of the surgical nurse will involve several stages, from basic education to advanced practice and leadership roles. To practice as a surgical nurse in Hong Kong, it is first necessary to complete a recognized nursing program, such as a Bachelor of Nursing. Upon graduation, it is normal practice to work in a surgical clinical setting as a staff nurse post-qualification, to gain foundational nursing experience. Post-registration experience will allow for further development of the essential nursing skills, patient care techniques, and gain more familiarity with surgical procedures. Nurses can pursue certification in surgical nursing, after a period working in surgical units or operating rooms, and this usually involves enrolment in a post-registration/postgraduate course.

Postgraduate studies for surgical nurses in Hong Kong provide a pathway for professional advancement and enhancing patient care. Surgical nurses may undertake a specified advanced practice program or pursue a general nursing master's degree; these types of educational programmed are offered by most of the higher education institutions in Hong Kong. Specialized programs in surgical nursing usually involve postgraduate academic study in conjunction with hands-on experience in advanced surgical nursing roles. The next level of career progression in surgical nursing maybe involve registration at advanced practice nurse (APN) level, which requires additional training and competency attainment in Hong Kong. To practice as an APN, and contribute significantly to patient reported outcomes, a surgical nurse is required to register with the Nursing Council of Hong Kong as an advanced practice nurse. With additional academic qualifications and surgical clinical experience, nurses may then consider other senior roles, such as nurse ward manager, clinical nurse specialist, nurse consultants, or as a nurse educators within the surgical setting. There may also be opportunities for surgically trained nurses in Hong Kong to pursue specific certifications to enhance their surgical expertise and professional standing within the local healthcare setting. This may include pursuing post-registration certification in wound care, provided by the Hong Kong Wound Care Association, or attain infection control certification from the Hospital Authority or other training institutions in Hong Kong. The Hospital Authority in Hong Kong also offers a wide variety of specialized training programs and continuing education qualifications for nurses who may be interested in developing a career pathway in surgical nursing. In relation to post-registration certification, it is important to note that while some specific nursing certifications in Hong Kong may be internationally recognized, others are tailored specifically for the Hong Kong hospital context. In summary, higher educational institutions in Hong Kong offer a wide range of educational programs and training opportunities for surgical nurses. Surgical nurses who engage in post-registration educational activities are likely to have better opportunities of promotion within the workplace, to positions like advanced nurse practitioner and beyond in the surgical setting.

Research

Nursing research involves systematic and scientific study of practice to develop knowledge to enhance nursing care and health promotion. In surgical nursing, research focuses on areas like improving patient reported outcomes, the quality of patient care, and occupational research. There are two main paradigms of nursing research design, quantitative and qualitative, each providing a distinct approach to the provision of evidence-based practice, leading to the improvement of the effectiveness of surgical nursing care.

Research is vital for surgical nurses; it has the potential to improve the quality of patient care, and it can directly influence professional growth and support advances within the nursing profession (Oster et al. 2020). Surgical nurses can use research findings to provide evidence-based care and promote positive outcomes for patients in their care and their family members. According to the American Nursing Association (2015), engaging and applying in research constitutes a fundamental aspect of professional nursing (Fowler 2015). As well as applying the findings of research studies which have been conducted by other nurse researchers, it is also important for surgical nurses to lead and participate in research projects and evidence-based practice studies, which have relevance within the surgical nursing arena (DeGrazia et al. 2019). Through the development and application of scientifically supported research methodology, surgical nurses can provide evidence-based care and improved patient outcomes. Application for nursing research can ensure that surgical nurses provide person-centered patient care, which is truly based on evidence and not on routine practice or intuition. Through engagement with research, surgical nurses can be empowered to contribute to the development of hospital policies and take on nursing leadership roles as nursing research can form the basis of surgical care protocols reducing clinical errors and optimizing nursing care. In this chapter, using different research methodology, examples are given of surgical nursing research studies that have led to safer more and effective patient surgical patient care. For example, in their systematic review and meta-analysis (Level 1 Evidence), Habtie et al. (2025) identified educational gaps and highlighted the impact of targeted training in relation to surgical site infection prevention among surgical nurses.

Quantitative Research Design

A randomized control trial (RCT) is a form of experimental study design that is used to assess the effectiveness of an intervention or treatment. This type of study can be viewed as the gold standard of clinical nursing research, enabling the determination of cause-and-effect relationships between interventions and health-related patient outcomes (Hariton and Locascio 2018). Taking an experimental approach, Fang et al. (2021) conducted an RCT and demonstrated that by using nurse-led pain relief models for patients undergoing abdominal surgery pain management can be improved in surgical patients. In another study, employing an RCT design, Aydal et al. (2023) highlighted the positive effect of nurse-led preoperative visits for surgical patients. They concluded that, through educational strategies, these preoperative visits greatly reduced patient reported levels of anxiety.

Another quantitative research methodology, observational study design, constitutes a type of research design that involves the nurse researcher monitoring interactions and processes within the surgical care setting. Generally, the observational researcher in surgical nursing care gathers research data on how surgical nursing care is provided and how surgical nurses can coordinate patient responses. Observational studies are important in surgical nursing research to provide greater understanding of real-world outcomes. There are several recognized types of observational research study design including case-control study, cohort study, and cross-sectional studies. Across each of these designs, the nurse researcher merely observes and records data, without manipulating any aspect of the study environment. In one prospective observational study, Taylor et al. (2018) reported that the implementation of electronic nurse LED assessment could greatly reduce time spent on assessment by surgical nurses, which potentially could enhance perioperative workflow. In another study, Choi et al. (2022) believed that surgical nursing care in conjunction with ERAS protocols can greatly improve patient reported clinical outcomes in the orthopedic setting. It is important to note that observational quantitative research studies tend to produce weaker evidence than experimental quantitative studies. RCT's generally provide much stronger evidence for surgical nurses, due mainly to their methodological strength with random assignment to treatment or control and other measures, which minimize the risk of bias and confounding variables.

These quantitative study designs, employing different research methods, demonstrate the importance of nursing research in the surgical sitting. The RCT gold standard clearly has the potential of impact, demonstrating the surgical nursing led innovations. From professional perspective, research also provides a strong empirical basis for the value of nursing leadership in the delivery of surgical care.

Qualitative Research Design

It is important that when considering the importance of research in surgical nursing care, that attention is also given to the vital role that qualitative research methods play. In surgical nursing, qualitative research methods approaches are incredibly important, as they enable researchers to gain a deeper insight into the human experience that cannot be captured through only employing quantitative methods. Qualitative research is valuable for uncovering factors that may lie behind surgical outcomes, potentially leading to improvement of quality surgical care. Generating deeper insights into clinical surgical problems through the exploration of patient's perspectives toward attitudes, beliefs, and interactions in the surgical setting can potentially uncover factors to enable improvement in quality of surgical care. Commonly used data collection methods for qualitative studies include the use of semi-structured interviews and focus groups. In one nursing qualitative study, Atthayasai et al. (2023) highlighted the importance of surgical nurses' role, in a multidisciplinary collaboration, when delivering advanced healthcare technological innovations to improve postsurgical pain management. By capturing the lived experience of these surgical patients, findings can potentially complement those findings from quantitative studies and make a significant contribution toward evidence-based practice within surgical nursing practice. By providing surgical nurses with greater comprehension of patient experiences, through the emotions and beliefs that may relate to having a surgical intervention, these could involve social, ethical, and cultural factors, which influence surgical clinical outcomes. As such, qualitative research can play an important role in the enhancement of communication in the delivery of person-centered surgical patient care.

Mixed Method Research Design

Taking a mixed method approach toward surgical research involves the combination of quantitative and qualitative research design to provide a more comprehensive overview to answer a research question. Taking a mixed method approach can leverage the strengths of both quantitative and qualitative research, and by integrating these methods, nurse researchers can gain a fuller picture than each individual approach alone. For example, this approach can help the nurse researcher to achieve generalizability through the quantitative element of a study and conceptualization from the qualitative element. Together, taking a mixed method approach can be helpful for the nurse research to understand complex clinical situations, where understanding both the "What?" (in quantitative approaches) and "Why?" (in qualitative approaches) is required. In Hong Kong, one surgical nursing mixed method study evaluated the effect of teamwork enhancement and quality improvement initiative on the surgical nursing work environment (Wai et al. 2021). For the quantitative phase, this study employed a quasi-experimental trial for the quantitative phase, which assessed the impact of an intervention and the qualitative phase involved focus groups interviews with nurses to explore their experience of interprofessional teamwork. Eaton et al. (2017) demonstrated the benefits of integrating the quantitative and qualitative phases of a research study using mixed methods, in the surgical nursing setting. Examining the holistic comprehension of pain management, they demonstrated that the combination of data types provided a more complete picture of pain management within surgical nursing practice.

Research plays a vital role in the surgical nursing specialty, guiding clinical practice, education, and patient reported outcomes. It underpins evidence-based practice and supports clinical decision-making; surgical nurses are greatly encouraged to actively engage, where possible, with research related to their surgical practice. Surgical nurses can take several approaches to become actively involved in research, including participation in institutional research projects, attending and presenting at academic conferences, designing and implementing QI initiatives, collaborating with academic institutions, and participating with professional organizations. In Hong Kong, the specialty of surgical nursing is provided by the Hong Kong College of Surgical Nursing (HKCSN), under the Hong Kong Academy of Nursing & Midwifery. In surgical nursing, the HKCSN promotes excellence, defines standards for advanced practice, and provides educational opportunities in surgical nursing. In summary, through active participation in research, surgical nurses can contribute to the advancement of surgical nursing practice and potentially improve patient related healthcare outcomes.

Research vs. Quality Improvement in Surgical Nursing

The World Health Organization (2018) emphasized the importance of quality improvement (QI) protocols in the surgical setting to enhance patient reported outcomes and reduce the risk of surgical complication. In surgical nursing, QI projects are closely associated with clinical nursing research. Whereas research aims to generate new knowledge, which is generalizable, quality improvement projects focus more upon improving existing processes or outcomes within a specific organization (Faiman 2021). These projects (QI) are usually more flexible than the systematic approaches required in research. Generally, QI projects are based on models, like the plan-do-study-act (PDSA) cycle; they tend not to pose additional risks for patients beyond routine care, as such; and they tend not to require ethical approval. One Hong Kong-based example of a successful quality improvement project is the surgical outcomes monitoring and improvement program. This QI program monitored surgical outcomes across 17 public hospitals in Hong Kong, by benchmarking the performance of surgical departments and identifying potential areas of improvement (patient reported surgical outcomes based upon preoperative risk factors), leading to improvement in emergency surgery outcomes. This project demonstrates a real example of a local QI project, which improved surgical nursing outcomes within the public hospital setting in Hong Kong. Quality improvement outcomes are usually conducted to be specific to the local surgical context and strive to enhance existing practices, rather than to develop new knowledge. Therefore, while research seeks to discover new knowledge, quality improvement projects tend to apply established interventions to improve local surgical care delivery. Both research and quality improvement are crucial in surgical nursing, but they do serve very different goals and frameworks within the healthcare provision.

What Is Evidence-Based Practice in Surgical Nursing?

Evidence-based practice is a vital aspect of surgical nursing; it involves the integration of the best available research evidence with clinicians' expertise and patients' values and can ensure the delivery of the highest quality personalized healthcare (Jadhav 2025). An example of an evidence-based practice protocol in surgical nursing in Hong Kong is the "Recommendations on Prevention of Surgical Site Prevention" issued by the Centre for Health Protection. This evidence is widely applied in hospitals, as a standard care bundle to reduce risk of infection in the surgical setting.

To fully integrate evidence-based practice into surgical nursing practice, there needs to be educational support professional development opportunities for nurses who have access to up-to-date research materials, including research databases and journals; availability of technological tools, like the clinical decision support systems, and sufficient budget allocation; and finally, and perhaps most importantly, the motivation and time from nursing staff to implement evidence-based practice activities in the surgical setting. Full implementation of evidence-based practice can only be placed when the nursing leadership in the surgical setting prioritizes the integration of evidence-based practice, providing the valuable time and resources that are required for the integration of evidence-based practice initiatives in surgical nursing. It is vitally important to stress that the implementation of evidence-based practice protocols can be very challenging for surgical nursing staff, who may either be resistant to the changes that may come with evidence-based practice initiatives or hesitant to change their established care practice and routines. For surgical nurses, it may be difficult to identify the most relevant information via research databases or gaining access to academic journals that provide the most up-to-date research findings. Lack of education and in-service training may provide another barrier to the implementation of evidence-based practice in the surgical setting. Gaps in education, such as the ability to appraise academic research papers, may lead to insufficient knowledge implementation of evidence-based practice. In addition, budgetary constraints may prevent the implementation of a new intervention or the development of a new technological innovation in the surgical setting. In summary, adopting the principles of evidence-based practice in the surgical clinical environment can lead to professional nursing development, enhance clinical decision-making, and lead to improvements in the overall quality of surgical nursing. Integrating evidence-based practice within the surgical environment has the potential to ensure that surgical nursing care is grounded in the best quality and most up-to-date scientific knowledge, enhancing surgical patient reported outcomes.

Conclusion

In this chapter, the importance of education and nursing within the surgical nursing specialty has been highlighted. To bridge the gap between theory and practice, more integration of the best research results into education-based practice is required. Strengthening research and education in surgical nursing is essential to prepare surgical nurses to meet the challenges they face in modern surgical care. Through research and education, surgical nurses can adapt to new challenges in healthcare delivery, like the application of technological innovations in the surgical environment.

References

American Nurses Association (2015) Code of ethics for nurses with interpretive statements. American Nurses Association.

Atthayasai J, Chatchumni M, Eriksson H, Mazaheri M (2023) Surgical nurses' perceptions of strategies to enhance pain management proficiency: a qualitative study. Nurs Rep 13(2):923–933. https://doi.org/10.3390/nursrep13020081

Audet LA, Bourgault P, Rochefort CM (2018) Associations between nurse education and experience and the risk of mortality and adverse events in acute care hospitals: a systematic review of observational studies. Int J Nurs Stud 80:128–146. https://doi.org/10.1016/j.ijnurstu.2018.01.007

Aydal P, Uslu Y, Ulus B (2023) The effect of preoperative nursing visit on anxiety and pain level of patients after surgery. J Perianesth Nurs 38(1):96–101. https://doi.org/10.1016/j.jopan.2022.05.086

DeGrazia M, Difazio RL, Connor JA, Hickey PA (2019) Building and sustaining a culture of clinical inquiry in a pediatric quaternary hospital. J Nurs Adm 49(1):28–34. https://doi.org/10.1097/NNA.0000000000000704

Eaton LH, Meins AR, Zeliadt SB, Doorenbos AZ (2017) Using a mixed methods approach to explore factors associated with evidence-based cancer pain management practice among nurses. Appl Nurs Res 37:55–60. https://doi.org/10.1016/j.apnr.2017.07.008

Faiman B (2021) Quality improvement projects and clinical research studies. J Adv Pract Oncol 12(4):360–361. https://doi.org/10.6004/jadpro.2021.12.4.1

Fang L, Chen L, Sun H, Xu Y, Jin J (2021) The effectiveness of using a nurse-led pain relief model for pain management among abdominal surgical patients: a single-center, controlled before-after study in China. Pain Manag Nurs 22(2):198–204. https://doi.org/10.1016/j.pmn.2020.08.004

Fowler MDM (2015) Guide to the code of ethics for nurses with interpretive statements: development, interpretation, and application, 2nd ed. American Nurses Association. Online available: https://www.homeworkforyou.com/static_media/uploadedfiles/1730667481_6267655__323.pdf. Accessed on 29 Sept 2025

Habtie TE, Feleke SF, Terefe AB, Alamaw AW, Abate MD (2025) Nurses' knowledge and its determinants in surgical site infection prevention: a comprehensive systematic review and meta-analysis. PLoS One 20(1):e0317887. https://doi.org/10.1371/journal.pone.0317887

Hariton E, Locascio JJ (2018) Randomised controlled trials—the gold standard for effectiveness research. BJOG 125(13):1716. https://doi.org/10.1111/1471-0528.15199

Jadhav VS (2025) Evidence-based practice in medical-surgical nursing. Int J Nurs Med Invest 10(3):31–36. https://innovationaljournals.com/index.php/ijnmi/article/view/1091

Oster CA, Ludwigson L, Lewis CL (2020) The value of "why": advancing clinical nurse led research. Appl Nurs Res 55:151289. https://doi.org/10.1016/j.apnr.2020.151289

Taylor SK, Andrzejowski JC, Wiles MD, Bland S, Jones GL, Radley SC (2018) A prospective observational study of the impact of an electronic questionnaire (ePAQ-PO) on the duration of nurse-led pre-operative assessment and patient satisfaction. PLoS One 13(10):e0205439. https://doi.org/10.1371/journal.pone.0205439

Vasilopoulos G (2024) Quality in contemporary surgical nursing. Clin Pract 14(4):1214–1215. https://doi.org/10.3390/clinpract14040096

Wai AK, Lam VS, Ng ZL, Pang MT, Tsang VW, Lee JJ, Wong JY (2021) Exploring the role of simulation to foster interprofessional teamwork among medical and nursing students: a mixed-method pilot investigation in Hong Kong. J Interprof Care 35(6):890–898. https://doi.org/10.1080/13561820.2020.1831451

World Health Organization (2018) Safe surgery saves life: the importance of surgical safety. WHO Press, Geneva Online available: https://www.who.int/docs/default-source/patient-safety/9789241598590-eng-checklist.pdf. Accessed on 29 Sept 2025

The Interplay of Leadership and Followership in Achieving Surgical Expertise

Siu-Ling Yuen and Alice Yip

Introduction: The Power of Partnership—Leading and Following in Nursing's Success

The efficacy of leadership is essential for fostering team cohesion and propelling organizational advancement (Gichuhi 2021; Zaccaro et al. 2018). Furthermore, within the specialized context of surgical nursing, skilled leadership is of utmost importance. Surgical nurses possess a unique and critical skill set, refined through rigorous training and experience (Magro et al. 2022). Their expertise encompasses not only advanced technical proficiency but also a nuanced understanding of patient care within the high-stakes surgical environment. Effective leadership capitalizes on this specialized knowledge, optimizing team performance and ensuring patient safety and positive surgical outcomes. In this process of continuous improvement, the role of the nursing leader is essential. Effective nursing leaders execute key leadership skills by providing clear direction to teammates, motivating their initiative for driving excellence, and guiding them toward organizational goals (Koivunen et al. 2024). Performance enhancement, both at the organizational and individual staff levels, is a continuous improvement process (Graban 2018). A strong leader in surgical nursing can effectively utilize the team's collective expertise, facilitating efficient communication, coordinating complex procedures, and fostering a culture of continuous improvement (Koivunen et al. 2024). This ongoing commitment to performance enhancement, driven by effective leadership, contributes significantly to both organizational growth and the delivery of high-quality patient care.

S.-L. Yuen (✉)
Hong Kong College of Surgical Nursing, Kowloon, HKSAR, China
e-mail: info@hkcsn.org.hk

A. Yip
School of Health Sciences, St. Francis University,
Tseung Kwan O, Hong Kong
e-mail: khyip@sfu.edu.hk

The momentum and sustainability of service enhancement within healthcare, particularly in surgical settings, are significantly influenced by the presence of effective followership (Koivunen et al. 2024). Strong followership, characterized by active engagement and commitment to shared goals, complements and strengthens nursing leadership. When followers actively participate in discussions and planning for improvement initiatives, their specific needs and perspectives can be addressed, fostering mutual understanding and enabling the development of appropriate strategies (Jordan et al. 2019; Koivunen et al. 2024; Lockwood 2017). Both the roles of nurse leader and follower are essential in driving the organization toward excellence. Leaders must possess the ability to make sound judgements and decisions that best serve the organization's developmental needs and promote overall enhancement (Harvey et al. 2020; Jordan et al. 2019; Lockwood 2017). Furthermore, a key responsibility of nurse leaders is fostering staff competency development to meet both organizational goals and individual professional growth aspirations (Koivunen et al. 2024). This includes cultivating effective followership skills among team members and strategically nurturing the leadership potential of promising individuals to cultivate the next generation of nurse leaders. This proactive approach to leadership development ensures a robust succession pipeline and contributes to the long-term health and vitality of the organization (George and Massey 2020). This collaborative approach, facilitated by a receptive and inclusive leadership style, is crucial for optimizing service delivery and achieving sustainable positive change within demanding surgical environment. The synergistic relationship between a skilled nurse leader and engaged followers creates a dynamic and responsive system capable of navigating the complexities of surgical care and driving continuous improvement (Graban 2018; Koivunen et al. 2024).

Learning Process: Bridging the Generational Gaps—Nursing Leader and Learning from Boomers to Alpha

Throughout childhood, obedience and deference to parental authority are emphasized (Chu et al. 2021). This pattern continues in the educational setting, where obedience to teachers is similarly expected (Tyler and Trinkner 2017). Upon entering the workforce, the emphasis shifts from formal instruction to mentorship by senior colleagues, often prioritizing received wisdom over experiential learning (Merriam and Baumgartner 2020). This pedagogical approach, rooted in limited historical access to resources and technology, reinforced this reliance on established authority figures (teachers, instructors, coaches, senior colleagues, and community members) as primary sources of knowledge (Ballantine et al. 2021). Prior to the widespread adoption of information technology, learning primarily occurred through interpersonal interactions, formal education, and textbook-based knowledge (Gibson and Smith 2018). Most teaching and learning were conducted through face-to-face transfer of knowledge and skills (Gherheş et al. 2021). As individuals mature and assume senior roles within their families or professional spheres, such as nursing, the expectation to instruct the next generation becomes prominent

(Currie et al. 2012). They are encouraged to adopt the roles of teacher, coach, trainer, instructor, and leader. This model frequently stresses the unidirectional dissemination of knowledge from senior to junior, rather than fostering a reciprocal learning environment where both generations benefit from shared experiences and insights. This traditional model contrasts with more contemporary approaches that emphasize critical thinking, independent inquiry, and learning through trial and error (Chu et al. 2021).

The contemporary nursing workforce embodies a complex interplay of generational perspectives, each shaped by distinct sociocultural and technological influences (Goh 2022). These generational differences manifest most prominently in preferred learning styles, presenting both opportunities and challenges for leadership development and continuing education within the profession. Understanding and accommodating these diverse learning preferences is crucial for fostering a dynamic and adaptable nursing workforce equipped to navigate the complexities of twenty-first century healthcare (Goh 2022; Zamiri and Esmaeili 2024). Furthermore, nurturing the next generation of competent staff and leaders is a fundamental responsibility of current leaders and senior nurses (Duffy 2022). This intergenerational mentorship is essential for ensuring the continued growth and success of healthcare organizations.

Nurses from the Baby Boomer [those born between 1946 and 1964] and Generation X [those born between 1965 and 1980] cohorts (Dimock 2019; Hisel 2020), who often occupy leadership roles, largely received their education and training within a formal, structured paradigm emphasizing face-to-face interaction (Zemke et al. 2013). Their engagement with professional development activities has traditionally been driven by a focus on career advancement and job security, reflecting the prevailing socioeconomic climate of their formative years (Fortes et al. 2022). This translates to a demonstrable proclivity toward established, in-person learning modalities.

Conversely, subsequent generations, encompassing Millennials [those born between 1981 and 2000] and Generation Z [members of Generation Z (those born after 1996) are now entering the workforce] (Dimock 2019; Hisel 2020), represent a paradigm shift in learning preferences (Chicca and Shellenbarger 2019; St-Denis 2016; Patten 2025). As digital natives, they exhibit an innate fluency in navigating the digital landscape, leveraging technology for knowledge acquisition, skill development, and collaborative learning experiences that transcend geographical boundaries (Sai et al. 2024). This inherent comfort with electronic learning modalities distinguishes them from their predecessors, highlighting the evolving role of technology in shaping professional development with nursing.

However, while embracing digital learning, these younger generations also place a significant emphasis on feedback mechanisms. This desire for validation, reassurance, and iterative improvement through mentorship and guidance emphasizes the enduring importance of intergenerational collaboration (Chicca and Shellenbarger 2019; St-Denis 2016). Creating opportunities for knowledge exchange and mentorship between experienced nurses and their younger counterparts is essential for fostering a supportive and inclusive learning environment. Understanding the worldview and learning styles of younger generations enhances communication, minimizes the generational gap, and facilitates the development of effective strategies for staff development and organizational growth (Fokeladeh et al. 2024).

Therefore, optimizing professional development within nursing requires a nuanced approach that acknowledges and integrates these diverse learning preferences (Tiago and Mitchell 2024; Zamiri and Esmaeili 2024). A blended learning strategy incorporating both traditional face-to-face instruction and innovative digital platforms is paramount (Anthony et al. 2019). This multifaceted approach not only caters to the specific needs of each generation but also fosters intergenerational understanding and collaboration, enriching the learning experience for all (Sai et al. 2024). Furthermore, embedding robust feedback mechanisms within both online and offline learning environments is crucial for supporting the growth and development of all nurses, regardless of generational affiliation. By recognizing and strategically addressing these intergenerational learning dynamics, nursing leadership can cultivate a culture of continuous learning, empowering nurses to thrive in the ever-evolving healthcare ecosystem (Ochis 2024).

Staff Development: The Enduring Importance of Nurse Leadership in Team Development and Organizational Performance

In the dynamic landscape of contemporary healthcare, effective nurse leaders are paramount for fostering high-performing teams and optimizing organizational outcomes (Chivaka 2024; da Silva 2025; McCauley and Palus 2021). Nurse leaders play a crucial role in cultivating a positive work environment, promoting professional development, and navigating the complexities of a multigenerational workforce (Cao et al. 2023; Kaiser and Westers 2018). This necessitates a nuanced understanding of individual learning styles, generational preferences, and the strategic implementation of innovative training methodologies.

Historically, nurse leaders have focused on building cohesive teams, developing team members' skills, and guiding them toward shred objectives (Cummings et al. 2021; McCauley and Palus 2021). This foundational approach remains essential, particularly in today's multigenerational workplace, which comprises individuals spanning from Baby Boomers to Generation Alpha [those born between 2010 and 2025] (Alzuman and Alzouman 2023; Hisel 2020; Höfrová et al. 2024). Each cohort presents unique characteristics, perspectives, and communication styles, requiring leaders to adapt their strategies accordingly (Hisel 2020). Effective leadership in this context involves recognizing, understanding, and respecting these generational differences to foster a sense of value and belonging among all team members (Hisel 2020). For instance, younger generations often gravitate toward hands-on, experiential learning and thrive on regular feedback that acknowledges their strengths and provides opportunities for improvement (Kennedy et al. 2021). This preference contrasts with traditional, lecture-based training models and emphases the need for innovative approaches to professional development.

Within daily practice, preceptors and mentors are strategically assigned to support the development of new generation of nurses. This structured approach facilitates clinical coach, skills enhancement, and effective debriefing, thereby fostering continuous learning and growth. Effective monitoring plays a critical role in this process, ensuring that new nurses receive the guidance and support necessary to establish a strong foundation in clinical practice (Duffy 2022). The preceptor-mentee relationship is particularly significant, providing a platform for individualized instruction, feedback, and professional socialization. As two studies from Vance (2022a, b) emphasizes, a robust mentoring culture within the workplace is essential for providing ongoing feedback, acknowledging strong performance, and fostering a sense of ownership among young professionals (Vance 2022a, b). This sense of ownership extends to performance improvement plans and career development plans, which should be established through open discussions that actively engage the individual in the planning process.

Furthermore, contemporary training methodologies are evolving to meet the specific needs and learning preferences of emerging generations. Simulation training, with its scenario-based learning and opportunities for direct feedback, has become a valuable tool for skills-based training and competency assessment (Decker et al. 2011; Di Leonardi et al. 2020; Keddington and Moore 2019; Nye 2021). Other innovative approaches, such as storytelling and situated clinical decision-making frameworks, offer engaging and interactive learning experiences that resonate with younger generations (Shorey et al. 2021; Thomas et al. 2020; Walker and Wilson 2024; Gillespie and Peterson 2009). These methods, coupled with effective preceptorship and mentorship, contribute to the development of well-rounded. Competent nurses prepared to meet the evolving demands of the healthcare landscape.

The impact of effective nurse leadership extends directly to organizational performance (Sorour et al. 2024). Well-trained, cohesive teams provide higher-quality patient care, enhance productivity through optimized workflows, and contribute to a positive work environment that fosters staff retention. Ultimately, nurse leaders shape the organizational culture by promoting values of collaboration, respect, and continuous improvement (Hisel 2020). Investing in nurse leadership development that encompasses these generational considerations is therefore essential for the future of healthcare. By embracing innovative training strategies and fostering a supportive learning environment, nurse leaders can empower the next generation of nurses to excel in their professional roles and contribute to a thriving healthcare system (Almutari and Almutairi 2023; Broome 2024).

Developing Leadership Potential: A Focus on Followership in Nursing

Mentorship plays a crucial role in leadership development by facilitating the newcomer's adaptation to role transitions and integration into the organizational culture (Bauer et al. 2025; Cai et al. 2021). This is achieved through active engagement of the developing leader in discussions and planning related to performance and service improvement. These interactive processes enhance the individual's understanding of the organizational culture, thereby facilitating both their adaptation and the formulation of individualized development plans (Viterouli et al. 2024). This approach fosters a more effective transition into leadership roles and contributes to the overall success of leadership development initiatives.

Engaging and empowering staff in service enhancement not only facilitates the gathering of valuable feedback for organizational improvement but also provides opportunities for staff to develop leadership skills (Islam et al. 2022; Park et al. 2022). Learning through engagement, a practice adopted by many organizations, enhances mutual understanding between leaders and followers, creating a reciprocal learning environment (Ahsan 2024; Fokeladeh et al. 2024; Mccarthy 2020; Nikolova et al. 2019; St-Denis 2016). The participatory processes of discussion and decision-making offer emerging leader's invaluable opportunities to observe effective leadership and followership in action, gaining practical experience in these critical areas (Day et al. 2021). This experiential learning complements the mentorship and coaching received in developing followership skills, further strengthening their potential for future leadership roles (Hisel 2020). A high-performing team requires both strong leadership and effective followership, and individuals demonstrating exemplary followership often possess the potential for future leadership roles (Einola and Alvesson 2021). Cultivating followership skills, therefore, serves as a valuable component of a comprehensive leadership development program (Dugan 2024).

Early engagement of emerging professionals in organizational projects fosters a sense of ownership and belonging based on self-determination theory (Lechler and Huemann 2024). The collaborative processes of discussion and planning inherent in project work provide valuable learning opportunities (Hisel 2020). Direct communication and open dialogue enable leaders to gain insights into the individual characteristics and perspectives of these future leaders, fostering a deeper understanding of their needs and aspirations (Ellinor and Girard 2023). This enhanced understanding facilitates the development of effective strategies for talent retention, professional development, and service enhancement. Simultaneously, early engagement provides emerging professionals with practical experience in teamwork and followership, cultivating essential skills that contribute to both individual and organizational success (Mazzetti and Schaufeli 2022). These experiences lay the foundation for their growth as future leaders within the organization.

While not every individual is destined for leadership, the vast majority can cultivate the qualities of an effective follower. Indeed, strong followership is essential for team efficacy and provides crucial support for leaders (Einola and Alvesson 2021). Moreover, effective followership is not merely a passive role; it is a fertile training ground for future leadership. A skilled follower, actively engaged and committed to the team's success, often demonstrates the potential for leadership (Mazzetti and Schaufeli 2022). Exceptional nursing leaders, in particular, recognize the inherent value of every team member, actively identifying and nurturing individual potential. By fostering a culture of growth and development, these leaders cultivate high-performing team and simultaneously cultivate the next generation of nursing leaders, ensuring the ongoing strength and vitality of the nursing profession, ultimately benefiting both the individual and the broader healthcare landscape (Barr and Nathenson 2022; Kartika 2024; Moloney et al. 2020; Yip et al. 2022; Zhu et al. 2021).

References

Ahsan MJ (2024) Cultivating a culture of learning: the role of leadership in fostering lifelong development. Learn Organ. https://doi.org/10.1108/TLO-03-2024-0099

Almutari MSW, Almutairi WSW (2023) Nursing leadership and management: theory, practice, and future impact on healthcare. Mohammed Saad Waslallah Almutari

Alzuman AS, Alzouman O (2023) Nurses' generational differences related to the workplace and leadership. Saudi J Nurs Health Care 6(8):252–271. https://doi.org/10.36348/sjnhc.2023.v06i08.003

Anthony B, Kamaludin A, Romli A, Raffei AFM, Nincarean A/L Eh Phon D, Abdullah A, Ming GL, Shukor NA, Nordin MS, Baba S (2019) Exploring the role of blended learning for teaching and learning effectiveness in institutions of higher learning: an empirical investigation. Educ Inf Technol 24:3433–3466. https://doi.org/10.1007/s10639-019-09941-z

Ballantine J, Stuber J, Everitt J (2021) The sociology of education: a systematic analysis. Routledge. https://doi.org/10.4324/9781003023715

Barr TL, Nathenson SL (2022) A holistic transcendental leadership model for enhancing innovation, creativity and well-being in health care. J Holist Nurs 40(2):157–168. https://doi.org/10.1177/08980101211024799

Bauer TN, Erdogan B, Ellis AM, Truxillo DM, Brady GM, Bodner T (2025) New horizons for newcomer organizational socialization: a review, meta-analysis, and future research directions. J Manag 51(1):344–382. https://doi.org/10.1177/01492063241277168

Broome ME (2024) Transformational leadership in nursing: from expert clinician to influential leader. Springer

Cai D, Liu S, Liu J, Yao L, Jia X (2021) Mentoring and newcomer well-being: a socialization resources perspective. J Manag Psychol 36(3):285–298. https://doi.org/10.1108/JMP-08-2019-0485

Cao H, Song Y, Wu Y, Du Y, He X, Chen Y, Wang Q, Yang H (2023) What is nursing professionalism? A concept analysis. BMC Nurs 22(1):34. https://doi.org/10.1186/s12912-022-01161-0

Chicca J, Shellenbarger T (2019) A new generation of nurses is here: strategies for working with generation Z. Am Nurse Today 14(2):48–51. Available as: https://link.gale.com/apps/doc/A584601977/AONE?u=anon~9a086054&sid=googleScholar&xid=a769e142

Chivaka R (2024) From a group of people to a well-functioning team: a transformative leadership model in healthcare. In: Multidisciplinary teamwork in healthcare. IntechOpen. https://doi.org/10.5772/intechopen.1005512

Chu SKW, Reynolds RB, Tavares NJ, Notari M, Lee CWY (2021) 21st century skills development through inquiry-based learning from theory to practice. Springer

Cummings GG, Lee S, Tate K, Penconek T, Micaroni SP, Paananen T, Chatterjee GE (2021) The essentials of nursing leadership: a systematic review of factors and educational interventions influencing nursing leadership. Int J Nurs Stud 115:103842. https://doi.org/10.1016/j.ijnurstu.2020.103842

Currie G, Lockett A, Finn R, Martin G, Waring J (2012) Institutional work to maintain professional power: recreating the model of medical professionalism. Organ Stud 33(7):937–962. https://doi.org/10.1177/0170840612445116

da Silva TMHR (2025) Navigating healthcare complexity: integrating business fundamentals into nursing leadership. In: Resiliency strategies for long-term business success. IGI Global, pp 145–168. https://doi.org/10.4018/979-8-3693-9168-6.ch006

Day DV, Riggio RE, Tan SJ, Conger JA (2021) Advancing the science of 21st-century leadership development: theory, research, and practice. Leadersh Q 32(5):101557. https://doi.org/10.1016/j.leaqua.2021.101557

Decker S, Utterback VA, Thomas MB, Mitchell M, Sportsman S (2011) Assessing continued competency through simulation: a call for stringent action. Nurs Educ Perspect 32(2)

Di Leonardi BC, Hagler D, Marshall DR, Stobinski JX, Welsh S (2020) From competence to continuing competency. J Contin Educ Nurs 51(1):15–24. https://doi.org/10.3928/00220124-20191217-05

Dimock M (2019) Defining generations: where millennials end and generation Z begins. Pew Research Center 17(1):1–7. Available at: https://www.pewresearch.org/fact-tank/2019/01/17/where-millennials-end-and-generation-z-begins/

Duffy JR (2022) Quality caring in nursing and health systems: implications for clinicians, educators, and leaders. Springer

Dugan JP (2024) Leadership theory: cultivating critical perspectives. Wiley

Einola K, Alvesson M (2021) When 'good'leadership backfires: dynamics of the leader/follower relation. Organ Stud 42(6):845–865. https://doi.org/10.1177/01708406198784722

Ellinor L, Girard G (2023) Dialogue: rediscover the transforming power of conversation. Crossroad Press

Fokeladeh HS, Montayre J, Stewart D (2024) International Council of Nurses 2025 Congress: nursing power to change the world. Int Nurs Rev 71(4):681–683. https://doi.org/10.1111/inr.13077

Fortes K, Latham CL, Vaughn S, Preston K (2022) The influence of social determinants of education on nursing student persistence and professional values. J Prof Nurs 39:41–53. https://doi.org/10.1016/j.profnurs.2021.11.011

George V, Massey L (2020) Proactive strategy to improve staff engagement. Nurse Lead 18(6):532–535. https://doi.org/10.1016/j.mnl.2020.08.008

Gherheș V, Stoian CE, Fărcașiu MA, Stanici M (2021) E-learning vs. face-to-face learning: analyzing students' preferences and behaviors. Sustainability 13(8):4381. https://doi.org/10.3390/su13084381

Gibson PF, Smith S (2018) Digital literacies: preparing pupils and students for their information journey in the twenty-first century. Inf Learn Sci 119(12):733–742. https://doi.org/10.1108/ILS-07-2018-0059

Gichuhi JM (2021) Shared leadership and organizational resilience: a systematic literature review. Int J Organ Leadersh 10(1):67–88

Gillespie M, Peterson BL (2009) Helping novice nurses make effective clinical decisions: the situated clinical decision-making framework. Nurs Educ Perspect 30(3):164–170

Goh AYS (2022) Learning journey: Conceptualising "change over time" as a dimension of workplace learning. Int Rev Educ 68(1):81–100. https://doi.org/10.1007/s11159-022-099432-2

Graban M (2018) Lean hospitals: improving quality, patient safety, and employee engagement. Productivity Press. https://doi.org/10.4324/9781315380827

Harvey G, Kelly J, Kitson A, Thornton K, Owen V (2020) Leadership for evidence-based practice—enforcing or enabling implementation? Collegian 27(1):57–62. https://doi.org/10.1016/j.colegn.2019.04.004

Hisel ME (2020) Measuring work engagement in a multigenerational nursing workforce. J Nurs Manag 28(2):294–305. https://doi.org/10.1111/jonm.12921

Höfrová A, Balidemaj V, Small MA (2024) A systematic literature review of education for Generation Alpha. Discov Educ 3(1):125. https://doi.org/10.1007/s44217-024-00218-3

Islam MN, Furuoka F, Idris A (2022) Transformational leadership and employee championing behavior during organizational change: the mediating effect of work engagement. South Asian J Bus Stud 11(1):1–19. https://doi.org/10.1108/SAJBS-01-2020-0016

Jordan Z, Lockwood C, Munn Z, Aromataris E (2019) The updated Joanna Briggs institute model of evidence-based healthcare. JBI Evid Implement 17(1):58–71. https://doi.org/10.1097/XEB.0000000000000155

Kaiser JA, Westers JB (2018) Nursing teamwork in a health system: a multisite study. J Nurs Manag 26(5):555–562. https://doi.org/10.1111/jonm.12582

Kartika ND (2024) The influence of transformational leadership on nurses' performances in Indonesia. Am J Phys Educ Health Sci 2(1):11–16. https://doi.org/10.54536/ajpehs.v2i1.2502

Keddington AS, Moore J (2019) Simulation as a method of competency assessment among health care providers: a systematic review. Nurs Educ Perspect 40(2):91–94. https://doi.org/10.1097/01.NEP.0000000000000433

Kennedy K, Leclerc L, Campis S (2021) Human-centered leadership in healthcare: evolution of a revolution. Morgan James Publishing

Koivunen K, Kaakinen P, Paeaetalo K, Mattila O, Oikarinen A, Jansson M, Mikkonen K, Põlkki T, Meriläinen M, Kääriäinen M, Holopainen A, Tuomikoski A, Kanste O (2024) Frontline nurse leaders' competences in evidence-based healthcare: a scoping review. J Adv Nurs 80(4):1314–1334. https://doi.org/10.1111/jan.15920

Lechler RC, Huemann M (2024) Motivation of young project professionals: their needs for autonomy, competence, relatedness, and purpose. Proj Manag J 55(1):50–67. https://doi.org/10.1177/87569728231195587

Lockwood C (2017) Applying theory informed global trends in a collaborative model for organizational evidence-based healthcare. J Korean Acad Nurs Adm 23(2):111–117. https://doi.org/10.11111/jkana.2017.23.2.111

Magro G, Dellai M, Notarnicola I (2022) Self-assessment the competencies of surgical and critical area nurses. A cross-sectional study. Acta Biomed Atenei Parmensis 93(6). https://doi.org/10.23750/abm.v93i6.13544

Mazzetti G, Schaufeli WB (2022) The impact of engaging leadership on employee engagement and team effectiveness: a longitudinal, multi-level study on the mediating role of personal-and team resources. PLoS One 17(6):e0269433. https://doi.org/10.1371/journal.pone.0269433

Mccarthy A (2020) Develop millennial leaders with generation collaboration. Am Nurse Today 15(12):5–7. Available as https://www.myamericannurse.com/wp-content/uploads/2020/12/an12-Millennial-1123.pdf

McCauley CD, Palus CJ (2021) Developing the theory and practice of leadership development: a relational view. Leadersh Q 32(5):101456. https://doi.org/10.1016/j.leaqua.2020.101456

Merriam SB, Baumgartner LM (2020) Learning in adulthood: a comprehensive guide. Wiley

Moloney W, Fieldes J, Jacobs S (2020) An integrative review of how healthcare organizations can support hospital nurses to thrive at work. Int J Environ Res Public Health 17(23):8757. https://doi.org/10.3390/ijerph17238757

Nikolova I, Schaufeli W, Notelaers G (2019) Engaging leader–engaged employees? A cross-lagged study on employee engagement. Eur Manag J 37(6):772–783. https://doi.org/10.1016/j.emj.2019.02.004

Nye C (2021) State of simulation research in advanced practice nursing education. Annu Rev Nurs Res 39(1):33–51

Ochis K (2024) Gen Z in work: a practical guide to engaging employees across the generations. Taylor & Francis

Park J, Han SJ, Kim J, Kim W (2022) Structural relationships among transformational leadership, affective organizational commitment, and job performance: the mediating role of employee engagement. Eur J Train Dev 46(9):920–936. https://doi.org/10.1108/EJTD-10-2020-01-0149

Patten YA (2025) Critical factors influencing generation Z registered nurses' professional socialization process: a grounded theory study. Nurse Educ Today 146:106514. https://doi.org/10.1016/j.nedt.2024.106514

Sai S, Sharma P, Gaur A, Chamola V (2024) Pivotal role of digital twins in the metaverse: a review. Digit Commun Netw. https://doi.org/10.1016/j.dcan.2024.12.003

Shorey S, Chan V, Rajendran P, Ang E (2021) Learning styles, preferences and needs of generation Z healthcare students: scoping review. Nurse Educ Pract 57:103247. https://doi.org/10.1016/j.nepr.2021.103247

Sorour MS, Abdelaliem SMF, Khattab SAK (2024) The impact of nurse managers' boundary spacing leadership on the relationship between nurses' work embeddedness and innovative work behaviors. BMC Nurs 23(1):1–14. https://doi.org/10.1186/s12912-024-02402-0

St-Denis V (2016) Meet the millennials: a new generation of nursing leaders. Can Nurse 112(6):28

Thomas A, Kuper A, Chin-Yee B, Park M (2020) What is "shared" in shared decision-making? Philosophical perspectives, epistemic justice, and implications for health professions education. J Eval Clin Pract 26(2):409–418. https://doi.org/10.1111/jep.13370

Tiago RDS, Mitchell A (2024) Integrating digital transformation in nursing education: best practices and challenges in curriculum development. In: Digital transformation in higher education, Leeds. Emerald Publishing Limited, pp 57–101. https://doi.org/10.1108/978-1-83608-424-220241004

Tyler TR, Trinkner R (2017) Why children follow rules: legal socialization and the development of legitimacy. Oxford University Press

Vance C (2022a) Mentoring the novice nurse. Promoting talent and potential. Nurs Econ 40(5). https://doi.org/10.62116/nec.2022.40.5.249

Vance C (2022b) Wherefore art thou, mentor? Nurs Econ 40(4):204–207

Viterouli M, Belias D, Koustelios A, Tsigilis N, Papademetriou C (2024) Time for change: designing tailored training initiatives for organizational transformation. In: Organizational behavior and human resource management for complex work environments. IGI global, pp 267–307. https://doi.org/10.4018/979-8-3693-3466-9.ch014

Walker S, Wilson J (2024) Using interactive theatre in education to explore how healthcare decision-making can cause inadvertent trauma. Ment Health Pract 27(5). https://doi.org/10.7748/mhp.2018.e1259

Yip YC, Yip KH, Tsui WK (2022) When rationing becomes inevitable in a pandemic: a discussion on the ethical considerations from public health perspective. Public Health Pract 4(100294):1–3. https://doi.org/10.1016/j.puhip.2022.100294

Zaccaro SJ, Green JP, Dubrow S, Kolze M (2018) Leader individual differences, situational parameters, and leadership outcomes: a comprehensive review and integration. Leadersh Q 29(1):2–43. https://doi.org/10.1016/j.leaqua.2017.10.003

Zamiri M, Esmaeili A (2024) Strategies, methods, and supports for developing skills within learning communities: a systematic review of the literature. Adm Sci 14(9):231. https://doi.org/10.3390/admsci14090231

Zemke R, Raines C, Filipczak B (2013) Generations at work: managing the clash of Boomers, Gen Xers, and Gen Yers in the workplace. Amacom

Zhu X, Kunaviktikul W, Sirakamon S, Abhicharttibutra K, Turale S (2021) A causal model of thriving at work in Chinese nurses. Int Nurs Rev 68(4):444–452. https://doi.org/10.1111/inr.12671

Enhancing Surgical Nursing: Innovative Approaches to Simulation Education and Practice

7

Chun-Kit Jacky Chan

Introduction

Clinical simulation has become an essential component of surgical nursing education and practice, offering a safe and controlled environment for nurses to develop critical skills, build competencies, and identify performance gaps. This pedagogical approach allows nurses to practice, trail, and refine their clinical techniques and workflow without risking patient safety, thereby fostering a deeper understanding of complex surgical procedures (Mariani et al. 2019; Yip et al. 2025). The integration of simulation into nursing practice not only enhances technical proficiency but also promotes important soft skills, such as teamwork and communication, which are vital in the high-stakes surgical interprofessional practice setting (Miller et al. 2020). By engaging in realistic scenarios, nurses are better prepared to face the challenges of real-life clinical situations, ultimately leading to improved patient outcomes (Kirkman et al. 2020). Furthermore, simulation provides opportunities for immediate feedback and debriefing, which are crucial for reflective learning and skill mastery (Fowler et al. 2021). As the field of surgical nursing continues to evolve, embracing innovative simulation practices can significantly enhance educational experience, ensuring that future nurses are equipped with the necessary tools to excel in their roles. This chapter will explore the design, evaluation, and future directions of surgical nursing which are different from other specialties. For how to run the simulation, this will not be covered by this chapter and the reader and refer to other simulation instructor courses.

C.-K. J. Chan (✉)
School of Nursing and Health Sciences, Hong Kong Metropolitan University, Kowloon, HKSAR, China
e-mail: jckchan@hkmu.edu.hk

Foundations of Surgical Nursing Simulation: Theoretical Framework Applied in Surgical Nursing Simulation

Experiential Learning Theory (ELT)

Experiential learning theory (ELT), developed by Kolb (1984), posits that knowledge is created through the transformation of experience. In the context of surgical nursing simulation, this theory underscores the importance of hands-on practice, where students are actively engaged in realistic clinical scenarios. This theory is the main pillar, which is used in all kinds of simulations. By participating in simulations, nurses undergo a cycle of concrete experience, reflective observation, abstract conceptualization, and active experimentation. This process allows them to apply theoretical knowledge in practice, thus bridging the gap between classroom instruction and real-world application. For instance, when students perform a simulated surgical procedure, they can reflect on their actions, receive immediate feedback, and adjust their techniques in subsequent simulations, leading to enhanced skill acquisition and confidence (Sitzmann 2011; Yip et al. 2025).

Constructivism

Constructivism is another classical and critical learning theory that informs simulation practices in surgical nursing. According to constructivist principles, learners actively construct their own understanding of the world through experiences and reflection (Bruner 1996). In surgical nursing simulations, students are encouraged to engage with scenarios actively, allowing them to explore, make decisions, and reflect on the consequences of their actions. This hands-on approach fosters deeper learning, as students are not merely passive recipients of information but active participants in their education. For example, when faced with a simulated surgical complication, students must apply critical thinking and problem-solving skills, leading to a more profound understanding of the complexities of patient care in surgical settings (Dewey 1938).

Proximal Social Learning Theory

Proximal social learning theory, rooted in Vygotsky's work, emphasizes the role of social interaction in learning. This theory is particularly relevant in surgical nursing education, where collaboration is critical. Simulation environments foster teamwork and communication among students, enabling them to learn from one another while performing tasks. In surgical settings, nurses often work in multidisciplinary teams, and simulation allows nursing students to practice these dynamics. Through peer interactions during simulations, students can share insights, challenge each other's assumptions, and collectively problem-solve, thus enhancing their learning experience (Palincsar 1998). The social aspect of learning in simulations reflects the realities of clinical practice, where effective communication and collaboration directly impact patient safety and outcomes.

The Concept of Community of Practice (CoP)

The concept of community of practice (CoP), introduced by Lave and Wenger (1991), further enriches the collaborative learning experience in surgical nursing simulation by Vygotsky in previous paragraph. CoP refers to a group of individuals who share a common interest and engage in collective learning. In the context of surgical nursing, simulation can create a CoP among students, educators, and practicing nurses. By interacting and sharing experiences within the simulation framework, students build a shared repertoire of knowledge and skills. This collaborative learning environment promotes a sense of belonging and encourages students to take ownership of their learning journey. As they engage with their peers and instructors, they develop not only technical competencies but also professional identities as future surgical nurses (Wenger 1998).

Competency-Based Education (CBE)/Entrusted Professional Activities (EPA) in Surgical Nursing Simulation

Competency-Based Education (CBE) and Entrustable Professional Activities (EPA) play a crucial role in enhancing surgical nursing simulation by providing a structured framework for training and assessment. CBE emphasizes equipping learners with specific competencies necessary for professional practice, while EPAs serve as units of professional practice that can be entrusted to trainees once they demonstrate sufficient competence. To effectively apply these concepts in surgical nursing, key competencies related to surgical procedures—such as sterile techniques, patient assessment, and communication—must be clearly defined. Subsequently, EPAs representing essential activities in surgical nursing, such as preparing for surgery, assisting in procedures, and providing postoperative care, should be developed to integrate knowledge, skills, and attitudes.

Realistic simulation scenarios that mimic actual surgical environments and procedures can then be designed, incorporating the identified competencies and EPAs to offer trainees hands-on experience. Assessment rubrics based on these EPAs will detail the criteria for evaluating performance during simulations, encompassing both technical and nontechnical skills like teamwork and communication. Trained evaluators can observe trainees, assessing their performance against these established rubrics, and provide constructive feedback that highlights strengths and areas for improvement. This iterative process encourages self-reflection among trainees, fostering continuous learning and skill enhancement.

Furthermore, the effectiveness of the CBE and EPA framework should be evaluated through data collection on trainee performance and outcomes post-simulation. Engaging stakeholders—such as nursing educators, clinical practitioners, and trainees—in this evaluation process will allow for a diverse range of perspectives and facilitate collaboration among educational institutions to share best practices. Ultimately, integrating CBE and EPA into surgical nursing simulation significantly enhances the training and readiness of nursing professionals, ensuring they are well-prepared to meet the complexities of surgical care.

Summary

The integration of these learning theories and model—Experiential Learning Theory, Constructivism, Proximal Social Learning Theory, Community of Practice, and Competency-Based Education (CBE)/Entrusted Professional Activities (EPA)—provides a robust framework for enhancing surgical nursing education through simulation. By creating an environment that emphasizes active participation, social interaction, collaborative learning, and critical reflection, nursing programs can better prepare nurses for the demands of clinical practice. The immersive nature of simulation not only builds technical skills but also fosters essential interpersonal competencies, such as communication and teamwork, which are vital in the surgical environment. Ultimately, this multifaceted approach to learning ensures that nurses are equipped with the knowledge, skills, and confidence necessary to excel in their roles and contribute to improved patient care outcomes in surgical settings.

Types of Simulation in Surgical Nursing and Differences Compare with Another Specialty

In surgical nursing, simulation serves as a powerful educational tool, encompassing two major types—simulation scenario and task training—that cater to different learning needs and objectives. High-fidelity whole scenario simulation immerses nurses in realistic, comprehensive environments, either in dedicated simulation labs or through in-situ simulation in operating theatre, where scenarios unfold in actual clinical settings, similar as other specialty nursing simulation. This type of simulation utilizes advanced technology, including lifelike mannequins and sophisticated monitoring systems, to replicate the complexities of patient care, allowing nurses to practice decision-making, teamwork, and critical thinking in a safe, controlled environment (Yip et al. 2025).

On the other hand, surgical nursing simulation has significant heavy portion on the task trainer's simulation compared with another specialty. Task trainers provide a focused approach for mastering specific procedural skills. These can range from simple manikins designed for hands-on practice of individual techniques—such as suturing or catheter insertion—to virtual platforms that simulate procedural tasks in a digital realm. Task trainers allow nurses to refine their skills through repetition and feedback, enhancing their confidence and competence in performing essential procedures before encountering real patients. Together, these types of simulation create a comprehensive learning experience that prepares surgical nurses for the challenges they will face in clinical practice.

One significant difference between surgical nursing simulation and simulations in other nursing specialties is that surgical nursing simulations typically involve role-playing scenarios with anesthesiologists and surgeons, which are rarely completed by surgical nurses alone. In contrast, nurses in other specialties may often conduct simulations independently (Pugh et al. 2017). Additionally, surgical nursing simulations frequently interact with the operating room environment and various medical devices, such as anesthetic machines, ECMO (extracorporeal membrane oxygenation), heart-lung machines, and numerous infusion pumps. These elements are less common in other specialties, which may not require such extensive interactions (Ziv et al. 2016). As a result, surgical nursing simulations are usually conducted in situ rather than in simulation labs to minimize setup time. However, this reliance on the operating room creates challenges related to the availability of time slots in the operating suite (McGaghie et al. 2010).

Measuring Outcomes in Surgical Nursing Simulation

Within surgical nursing, validated psychometric instruments exist for the assessment of team performance and outcomes. The following table excludes tools designed for general teamwork measurement or those specific to other specialties such as resuscitation, although numerous examples can be found in the literature. Table 7.1 highlights several commonly employed instruments:

Table 7.1 Common instruments in surgical nursing simulation

Scale	Author	Scale	Content	Assessment target
Oxford NOTECHS II (nontechnical skills)	Fleetwood et al. (2018), United States of America	5 points	4 domains: Leadership and management, teamwork and cooperation, problem solving and decision making, and situation awareness	Individuals
NOTSS (nontechnical skills for surgeons)	Yule et al. (2008), United Kingdom	4 points	Situation awareness, decision making, communication and teamwork, leadership	Individuals
RAS-NOTECHS (robotic-assisted surgery (RAS))	Schreyer et al. (2022), Germany	4 points	Situation awareness, decision making, communication and teamwork, leadership	Individuals
ANTS (anesthetists' nontechnical skills)	Fletcher et al. (2003), United Kingdom	4 points	Task management, situational awareness, teamwork, and decision making	Individuals
OTAS (observational teamwork assessment for surgery)	Undre et al. (2006), United Kingdom	7 points	Communication, leadership, cooperation, coordination, and monitoring	Whole team
SO-DIC-OR (simultaneous observation of distractions and communication in the operating room)	Seelandt et al. (2014), Switzerland	Event coding	Teamwork/communication categories—case relevant communication, teaching, leadership, problem solving, case-irrelevant communication, laughter, tension, and communication with visitors	Whole team

Common Challenges in Surgical Nursing Simulation and Potential Solution

Surgical nursing simulation presents a range of challenges that can impede the effectiveness of training programs aimed at enhancing the skills and competencies of nursing professionals. These challenges include the need for realistic simulation environments, the integration of multidisciplinary team training, and the development of validated assessment tools to evaluate the effectiveness of simulation-based education (Yip et al. 2025).

One significant challenge in surgical nursing simulation is the creation of realistic scenarios that accurately reflect the complexities of clinical practice. As noted by John and Marath, there is a pressing need to improve existing simulation curricula by replicating real-life conditions encountered in nursing facilities (John and Marath 2022). This realism is crucial for preparing nurses to respond effectively to clinical deterioration, as highlighted in the meta-analysis by Orique and Phillips, which emphasizes the importance of simulation in equipping nurses with the necessary skills for competent patient care (Orique and Phillips 2017). Furthermore, Lewis et al. support this notion by demonstrating that simulation training for acute care nurses leads to improved patient safety outcomes, reinforcing the necessity of realistic training environments (Lewis et al. 2019).

Another challenge is the effective integration of multidisciplinary team training within surgical simulations. The literature indicates that teamwork and communication are critical components of successful surgical outcomes. Tan et al. discuss how multidisciplinary team simulation enhances not only technical skills but also non-technical skills such as communication and teamwork dynamics (Tan et al. 2013). This is echoed by the findings of Vigo et al., which show that structured training protocols for surgical teams, including nurses, can lead to improved operational efficiency and reduced costs (Vigo et al. 2021). Thus, fostering a collaborative learning environment through simulation can address the complexities of surgical care and improve overall patient outcomes.

To address the challenges faced in surgical nursing simulation training, implementing mandatory and protected time for nurses to participate in simulation sessions is essential. This approach can help overcome time constraints, ensuring consistent participation and engagement in training activities (McGaghie et al. 2010). Additionally, incorporating nontechnical skills training—such as assertiveness and systematic responses to emergencies—into existing programs is crucial, as these skills have been shown to enhance performance in real clinical situations (Kirkpatrick et al. 2020). By fostering both technical and nontechnical competencies, surgical nursing training can become more comprehensive and effective, ultimately leading to improved patient outcomes.

Future Directions: Virtual Reality

Virtual reality (VR) simulations have demonstrated significant enhancements in training outcomes for surgical procedures, improving procedural times, task completion rates, and accuracy while also receiving positive user ratings and showcasing cost-effectiveness (Mao et al. 2021; Huang et al. 2019; Ziv et al. 2016). This cutting-edge technology offers a safe and effective platform for nursing students, significantly enhancing their efficacy, attitudes, and confidence in perioperative settings (Siah et al. 2022; Kneebone et al. 2016). The integration of advanced technologies is set to revolutionize simulation in surgical nursing. High-fidelity mannequins equipped with sensors and artificial intelligence (AI) will facilitate more realistic scenarios, providing real-time feedback and adaptive learning experiences. Moreover, the increasing adoption of VR and augmented reality (AR) technologies allows nurses to practice complex procedures in immersive environments. These innovations can simulate rare or high-risk situations that are infrequently encountered in clinical practice, thereby enhancing overall preparedness (Becker et al. 2021).

Personalized Learning Experiences with Artificial Intelligence

Personalized learning experiences are becoming increasingly critical in simulation-based education. By utilizing data analytics, educators can tailor simulation scenarios to address the unique needs of individual learners, enabling nurses to develop competencies at their own pace. This approach not only highlights specific areas for improvement but also provides targeted practice opportunities, significantly enhancing the effectiveness of training programs (Cook et al. 2019). Furthermore, the integration of artificial intelligence (AI) and machine learning algorithms is revolutionizing the assessment of surgical expertise by analyzing extensive datasets generated from virtual reality (VR) simulations, offering deeper insights into psychomotor performance (Winkler-Schwartz et al. 2019; Gonzalez et al. 2020; MacKenzie et al. 2021). Tools like the Virtual Operative Assistant deliver automated feedback that effectively bridges the gap between novice and expert proficiency (Mirchi et al. 2020; Agarwal et al. 2020). Ultimately, the incorporation of VR and AI technologies not only aids in the acquisition of clinical psychomotor skills but also results in educational outcomes that are comparable to, or even superior to, those achieved through traditional training methods (Kneebone et al. 2016; Ziv et al. 2016). These advanced technologies support a range of educational objectives, including procedural skills training, emergency response training, soft skills development, and enhancement of psychomotor skills.

Conclusion

In conclusion, the integration of clinical simulation into surgical nursing education represents a transformative approach to training, equipping nurses with the essential technical and interpersonal skills necessary for effective practice. By leveraging theories such as Experiential Learning, Constructivism, and Proximal Social Learning, simulation fosters an immersive learning environment that encourages active participation, critical thinking, and collaborative problem-solving. This pedagogical framework not only enhances technical proficiency but also promotes vital soft skills like communication and teamwork, which are critical in high-pressure surgical settings.

Moreover, the distinction between surgical nursing simulation and other specialties highlights the unique challenges and opportunities within this field. The reliance on task trainers and high-fidelity simulations enables nurses to master specific skills while simulating the complexities of real-life clinical scenarios. However, challenges remain, including the need for realistic environments and effective multidisciplinary team training. Addressing these issues through structured training protocols and dedicated time for simulations can significantly enhance educational outcomes and ultimately improve patient safety.

Looking ahead, the incorporation of advanced technologies such as VR and AI promises to further enrich surgical nursing education. These innovations provide personalized learning experiences that cater to individual competencies and enhance the realism of simulated scenarios. As the field evolves, embracing these technologies will be crucial for preparing future surgical nurses to navigate the complexities of patient care effectively. Through continuous adaptation and improvement of simulation practices, surgical nursing education can ensure that graduates are not only proficient in their technical skills but also adept in the collaborative, high-stakes environment of surgical care, leading to better patient outcomes.

References

Agarwal M, Fattahi T, Tsai T (2020) The virtual operative assistant: bridging the gap in surgical training. Surg Endosc 34(4):1720–1726. https://doi.org/10.1007/s00464-019-06977-0

Becker K, Henneman EA, Hutton MJ (2021) The impact of simulation on nursing education: a review of the literature. Nurse Educ Today 97:104677. https://doi.org/10.1016/j.nedt.2020.104677

Bruner JS (1996) The process of education. New York: Vintage

Cook DA, Hatala R, Brydges R, Zendejas B, Hamstra SJ (2019) Technology-enhanced simulation for health professions education: a systematic review and meta-analysis. JAMA J Am Med Assoc 302(12):1330–1338. https://doi.org/10.1001/jama.2019.11546

Dewey J (1938) Experience and education. New York: Macmillan Publishing Company

Fleetwood VA, Veenstra B, Wojtowicz A, Kerchberger J, Velasco J (2018) Communication through simulation: developing a curriculum to teach interpersonal skills. Surgery 164(4):802–809. https://doi.org/10.1016/surg.2018.05.037

Fletcher G, Flin R, McGeorge P, Glavin R, Maran N, Patey R (2003) Anaesthetists' Non-Technical Skills (ANTS): evaluation of a behavioural marker system. Br J Anaesth 90(5):580–588. https://doi.org/10.1093/bja/aeg112

Fowler DM, Barlow J, Coyle R (2021) Enhancing learning through simulation: a comprehensive approach for nursing students. Nurse Educ Today 99:104794

Gonzalez R, McAuley J, Kahn D (2020) The role of artificial intelligence in surgical education: a comprehensive review. J Surg Educ 77(6):1343–1350. https://doi.org/10.1016/j.jsurg.2020.03.002

Huang MH, Liu CH, Wu YT (2019) The effectiveness of virtual reality simulation in improving nursing students' clinical performance: a meta-analysis. Nurse Educ Today 82:63–70. https://doi.org/10.1016/j.nedt.2019.08.006

John B, Marath U (2022) Simulation in pediatric nursing education: are there enough evidence for future practice? IP J Paediatr Nurs Sci 4(4):121–126. https://doi.org/10.18231/j.ijpns.2021.026

Kirkman MA, Chavda R, Ghosh R (2020) The impact of simulation-based training on surgical nursing competencies. J Surg Educ 77(2):267–273

Kirkpatrick AW, Boulanger BR, Sutherland FR (2020) Non-technical skills for surgical teams: a review of the literature. Can J Surg 63(2):E99–E105. https://doi.org/10.1503/cjs.005620

Kneebone R, Scott W, Darzi A (2016) The role of simulation in surgical education: a review. J Surg Res 206(1):1–10. https://doi.org/10.1016/j.jss.2016.05.007

Kolb DA (1984). Experiential learning: Experience as the source of learning and development. Englewood Cliffs, NJ: Prentice-Hall

Lave J, Wenger E (1991) Situated learning: Legitimate peripheral participation. Cambridge: Cambridge University Press.

Lewis K, Ricks TN, Rowin A, Ndlovu C, Goldstein LA, McElvogue C (2019) Does simulation training for acute care nurses improve patient safety outcomes: a systematic review to inform evidence-based practice. Worldviews Evid-Based Nurs 16(5):389–396. https://doi.org/10.1111/wvn.12396

MacKenzie CF, Zhang C, Miller J (2021) Machine learning algorithms for performance assessment in surgical training: a systematic review. Surg Endosc 35(7):3542–3551. https://doi.org/10.1007/s00464-020-08254-0

Mao R, Lan L, Kay J, Lohre R, Ayeni O, Goel D, Sa D (2021) Immersive virtual reality for surgical training: a systematic review. J Surg Res 268:40–58. https://doi.org/10.1016/j.jss.2021.06.045

Mariani B, Cantrell M, Barlow J (2019) Simulation in nursing education: the role of the debriefing process. Nurs Educ Perspect 40(4):226–231

McGaghie WC, Issenberg SB, Petrusa ER, Scalese RJ (2010) Medical education powered by simulation technology. Med Teach 32(8):663–668. https://doi.org/10.3109/0142159X.2010.501114

Miller M, Fenton J, McGowan J (2020) Teamwork and communication in surgical nursing: the role of simulation training. Am J Surg 219(5):1016–1021

Mirchi N, Bissonnette V, Yilmaz R, Ledwos N, Winkler-Schwartz A, Maestro R (2020) The virtual operative assistant: an explainable artificial intelligence tool for simulation-based training in surgery and medicine. PLoS One 15:e0229596. https://doi.org/10.1371/journal.pone.0229596

Orique SB, Phillips LJ (2017) The effectiveness of simulation on recognizing and managing clinical deterioration: meta-analyses. West J Nurs Res 40(4):582–609. https://doi.org/10.1177/0193945917697224

Palincsar AS (1998) Social constructivist perspectives on teaching and learning. In An introduction to Vygotsky. New York: Routledge

Pugh D, Cavalcanti RB, Halman S, Ma IWY, Mylopoulos M, Shanks D, Stroud L (2017) Using the entrustable professional activities framework in the assessment of procedural skills. J Grad Med Educ 9(2):209–214. https://doi.org/10.4300/JGME-D-16-00282.1

Schreyer J, Koch A, Herlemann A, Becker A, Schlenker B, Catchpole K, Weigl M (2022) RAS-NOTECHS: validity and reliability of a tool for measuring non-technical skills in robotic-assisted surgery settings. Surg Endosc 36:1916–1926. https://doi.org/10.1007/s00464-021-08474-2

Seelandt JC, Tschan F, Keller S, Beldi G, Jenni N, Kurmann A, Candinas D, Semmer NK (2014) Assessing distractors and teamwork during surgery: developing an event-based method for direct observation. BMJ Qual Safety 23(11):918–929. https://doi.org/10.1136/bmjqs-2014-002860

Siah R, Xu P, Teh C, Kow A (2022) Evaluation of nursing students' efficacy, attitude, and confidence level in a perioperative setting using virtual-reality simulation. Nurs Forum. https://doi.org/10.1111/nuf.12783

Sitzmann T (2011) A meta-analytic examination of the instructional effectiveness of computer-based simulation games. Personnel psychology 64(2):489–528. https://doi.org/10.1111/j.1744-6570.2011.01190.x

Tan SB, Pena G, Altree M, Maddern GJ (2013) Multidisciplinary team simulation for the operating theatre: a review of the literature. ANZ J Surg 84(7–8):515–522. https://doi.org/10.1111/ans.12478

Undre S, Healey AN, Darzi A, Vincent CA (2006) Observational assessment of surgical teamwork: a feasibility study. World J Surg 30:1774–1783. https://doi.org/10.1007/s00268-005-0488-9

Vigo F, Egg R, Schoetzau A, Montavon C, Brezak M, Heinzelmann-Schwarz V, Kavvadias T (2021) An interdisciplinary team-training protocol for robotic gynecologic surgery improves operating time and costs: analysis of a 4-year experience in a university hospital setting. J Robot Surg 16(1):89–96. https://doi.org/10.1007/s11701-021-01209-4

Wenger E (1998) Communities of practice: Learning, meaning, and identity. New York: Cambridge University Press

Winkler-Schwartz A, Bissonnette V, Mirchi N, Ponnudurai N, Yilmaz R, Ledwos N, Siyar S, Azarnoush H, Karlik B, Maestro R (2019) Artificial intelligence in medical education: best practices using machine learning to assess surgical expertise in virtual reality simulation. J Surg Educ 76(6):1681–1690. https://doi.org/10.1016/j.jsurg.2019.05.015

Yip A, Yip J, Tsui Z, Chan CKJ (2025) Standing strong: simulation training and the emotional resilience of healthcare providers during COVID-19. COVID 5(6):92. https://doi.org/10.3390/covid5060092

Yule S, Flin R, Maran N, Rowley D, Youngson G, Paterson-Brown S (2008) Surgeons' non-technical skills in the operating room: reliability testing of the NOTSS behavior rating system. World J Surg 32:548–556. https://doi.org/10.1007/s00268-007-9320-z

Ziv A, Wolpe PR, Small SD, Glick S (2016) Simulation-based medical education: an ethical imperative. Acad Med 81(8):771–778. https://doi.org/10.1097/ACM.0b013e3181e9b1d0

Exploring New Approaches and Techniques in Urology Nursing Care: Local Experience of Advancements and Innovations for Improved Patient Outcomes

8

Ka-Lok Lui, Alice Yip, Ka-Hing Chan, Yeung-Wan Sy, and Wing-Chi Kung

Introduction

Since prehistoric times, our understanding of urology has rapidly expanded. Thousands of years later, armed with an increased knowledge of anatomy and medicine, urological practice is at a stage where much of the effort is focused on producing technology that enables a minimally invasive, individualized, and targeted approach to treating disease. Urology nurse specialists provide the opportunity for innovative solutions in the daily management of patients. Within the context of a surgical specialty combining both medical and surgical management needs, these nurses are able to offer creative approaches to patient care. They have the opportunity to integrate patient-centered problem-solving skills with the specific needs of diverse urological patients. As a dynamic, adaptable, and vital complement to the care management of urological patients, these nurses can enhance access, manage chronic urological conditions, and improve patient satisfaction (Lajiness and Quallich 2016; Quallich and Lajiness 2020). As the shortage of urologists persists concurrently with the continued aging of the population requiring greater urological care services, the role of urology nurse specialists is becoming increasingly important.

It is hoped that this chapter provides insight into the rapidly expanding potential for urology nurse specialists, as many go on to specialize in urologic oncology, sexual dysfunction, incontinence, or stone disease. The intent of this chapter is to

K.-L. Lui (✉) · K.-H. Chan · Y.-W. Sy · W.-C. Kung
Hong Kong East Cluster Urology Team, Hospital Authority, Chai Wan, HKSAR, China
e-mail: luikl01@ha.org.hk; chankh02@ha.org.hk; syw086@ha.org.hk; kwc485@ha.org.hk

A. Yip
School of Health Sciences, St. Francis University,
Tseung Kwan O, Hong Kong
e-mail: khyip@sfu.edu.hk

"

serve as a guide, offering directions on discrete areas of urology care and providing resources to further cultivate both knowledge and skills from an advanced practice perspective. This chapter seeks to highlight the substantial potential of urology nurse specialists by presenting findings from retrospective studies conducted within clinical settings in Hong Kong. The subsequent discussion of urology reports aims to illustrate how these specialists contribute to delivering high-quality, cost-effective care for urology patients.

Digital Video Camera for Teaching Clean Intermittent Self-Catheterization in Female Patients

Clean intermittent self-catheterization (CISC) has been utilized as one of the primary alternatives for managing patients with voiding dysfunction (Hentzen et al. 2019). However, CISC is not a procedure to be undertaken without due consideration. CISC can cause stress, anxiety, and depression, particularly in female patients, as self-visualization of the urethral meatus may not be as straightforward as anticipated (Wang et al. 2021). To facilitate access to the urethral meatus during CISC, a digital video camera was utilized to project the view onto a digital screen display (Fig. 8.1).

Study Sharing: I

Between December 2016 and December 2017, 25 female patients participated in a study, with 13 in the digital video arm and 12 in the mirror arm. The mean age was 58.4 years. Regarding ease of use, the mean score was 32.5/40 in the digital video arm compared to 29.9/40 in the control group ($P > 0.05$). For ease of catheter insertion, the mean score was 4.1/5 in the digital video arm versus 3.3/5 in the control arm ($P < 0.05$). The mean score for patient confidence to implement CISC was 4/5 in the digital video arm compared to 3.3/5 in the control arm ($P < 0.05$). At the

Fig. 8.1 A digital video camera with a digital screen display

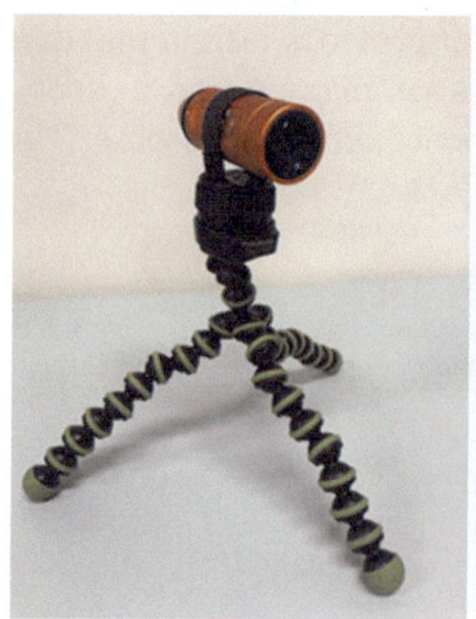
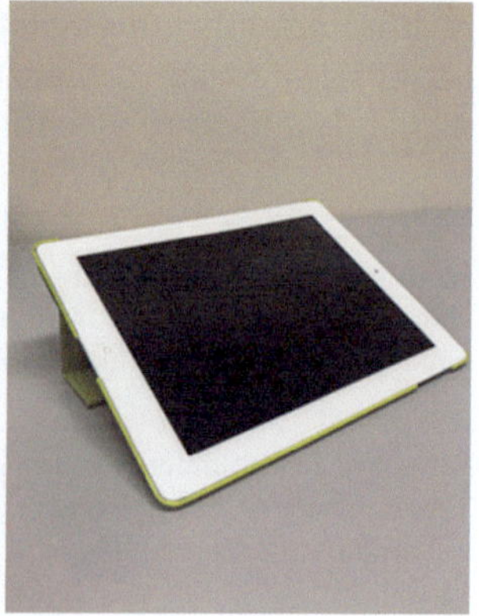

2-week follow-up, there were no complications such as bleeding or symptomatic lower urinary tract infection.

CISC in female patients can be complex, as many patients may not be able to perform it properly (Newman et al. 2018). Additional difficulties arise from problems such as decreased visual acuity, decreased motor dexterity, and preconceptions about manipulating their genitals. The use of a digital video camera in educating female patients on CISC leads to an improved understanding of their anatomy, increased patient perceptions, and greater motivation to learn CISC correctly.

The Effectiveness of Percutaneous Tibial Nerve Stimulation Therapy for Patients with Overactive Bladder Syndrome

Overactive bladder syndrome (OAB) is a highly prevalent condition, yet not all patients exhibit adequate responses to first-line (behavioral therapies) and second-line (pharmacological management) treatments (Corcos et al. 2017; Scarneciu et al. 2021). Percutaneous tibial nerve stimulation (PTNS) therapy has been proposed as a different, minimally invasive technique for treating OAB. PTNS therapy is a peripheral type of neuromodulation that utilizes electrical stimulation via a percutaneous needle to stimulate the posterior tibial nerve at the ankle (Peters et al. 2010; Ramírez-García et al. 2019) (Fig. 8.2).

Study Sharing: II

Between June 2014 and June 2019, 76 patients (13 males, 63 females) were recruited for the retrospective study in clinical settings. The mean age was 57 years (range 27–83). The results demonstrated a significant decrease in urinary frequency and urgency following PTNS therapy. The mean daytime voids decreased from 14.21 to

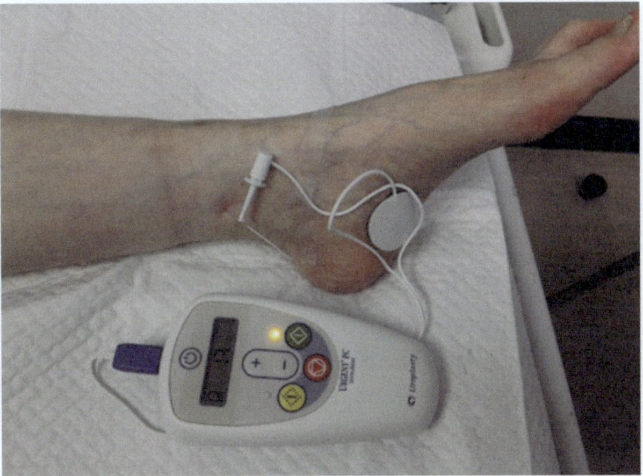

Fig. 8.2 Percutaneous tibial nerve stimulation therapy performed on the ankle of a patient

7.13 ($P < 0.05$). The mean number of nocturnal voids decreased from 3.12 to 2.13 ($P = 0.05$). The number of urge incontinence episodes per day significantly decreased from 2.75 to 1.30 ($P < 0.05$). The mean maximal voiding capacity increased from 110 to 223 ml ($P < 0.05$), and the mean minimal voiding capacity increased from 32 to 106 ml ($P < 0.05$). The mean overactive bladder symptom score (OABSS) decreased from 14.0 to 9.0 ($P < 0.05$), the mean urogenital distress inventory (UDI-6) score decreased from 8.5 to 6.5 ($P < 0.05$), and the mean incontinence impact questionnaire (IIQ-7) score decreased from 14.7 to 12.6 ($P < 0.05$). There were no complications or adverse events during or after PTNS therapy.

Patients expressed overall satisfaction with the treatment outcomes. There was a significant reduction in urge incontinence episodes, which adversely impacted patients' quality of life. Overall, the results were encouraging and support the recommendation of PTNS therapy as a treatment option for OAB patients who have failed first- and second-line therapies.

Management of Erectile Dysfunction with Low-Intensity Extracorporeal Shock Wave Therapy

The current nonsurgical treatment options for organic erectile dysfunction (ED) predominantly consist of oral phosphodiesterase type 5 inhibitors, intracavernosal injections of vasodilating agents, and/or vacuum pump devices (Argiolas et al. 2023; Madeira et al. 2021; Yafi et al. 2016). These treatments are effective and reasonably safe, with rare adverse effects. However, they share a major limitation in that they do not improve the underlying physiology of the erectile mechanism. These therapies are generally taken on-demand prior to sexual activity; thus, their effect is time-limited (Atallah et al. 2021).

Shock wave therapy has been widely utilized in extracorporeal shock wave lithotripsy (ESWL) (Lawler et al. 2017; Rola et al. 2022). It was modified and applied as low-intensity extracorporeal shock wave therapy (ESWT) with demonstrated efficacy in numerous studies for the treatment of ED (Adeldaeim et al. 2021; Clavijo et al. 2017; Man and Li 2018; Lu et al. 2017).

Study Sharing: III

Between 2015 and 2017, 94 male patients aged 42–80 years (mean 58.7) with ED of approximately 44 months' duration were recruited for a retrospective study of ESWT. During the study period, no other treatments for ED were administered. ESWT sessions lasting 13 min were well tolerated without anesthesia or side effects. Patients were encouraged to engage in sexual intercourse to reflect the potential efficacy of ESWT. The Sexual Health Inventory for Men (SHIM) score improved by 53.6% (11–16.9) at 4 weeks ($P < 0.05$), 48.1% (11–16.3) at 16 weeks ($P < 0.05$),

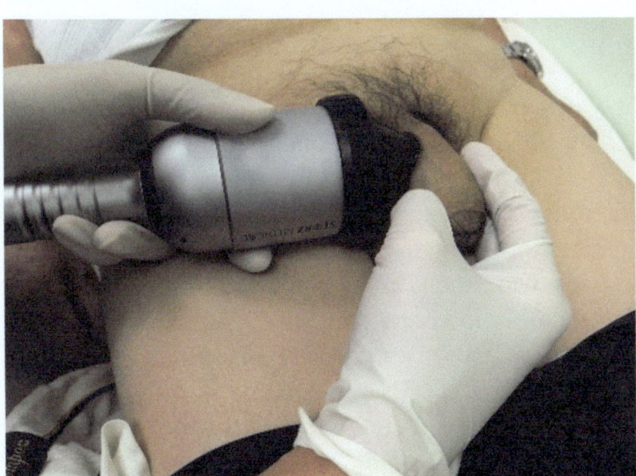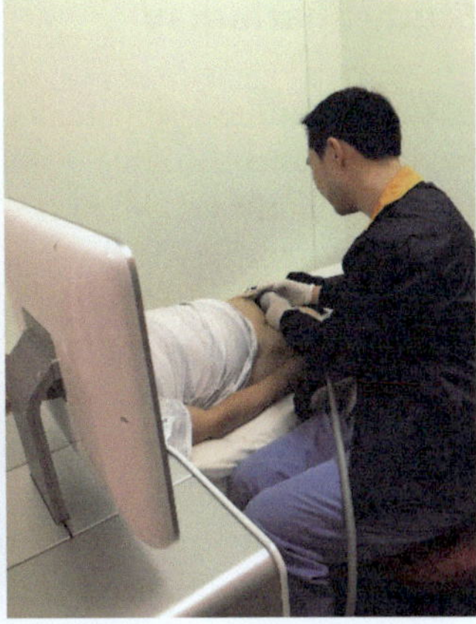

Fig. 8.3 A nurse specialist applied low-intensity extracorporeal shock wave therapy to a male patient with erectile dysfunction

and 43.6% (11–15.8) at 28 weeks ($P < 0.05$) following ESWT. Additionally, the Erection Hardness Score (EHS) improved by 45% (2–2.9) at 4 weeks ($P < 0.05$), 16 weeks ($P < 0.05$), and 36% (2–2.72) at 28 weeks ($P < 0.05$) after ESWT.

Extracorporeal shock wave therapy represents a new treatment option for patients with ED (Fig. 8.3). It is an effective intervention, especially for patients contraindicated for medical therapy (Adeldaeim et al. 2021; Bocchino et al. 2023). The role of the nurse specialist is critical in facilitating the process to ensure patient compliance and acceptance.

Nursing Perspectives on Management of Stent Irritative Symptoms: Initial Experience with Removal of Magnetic Ureteral Double-J Stents

Self-retaining ureteral stents are frequently used to relieve or prevent obstruction of the upper urinary tract after urinary stone surgery (Ramachandra et al. 2020). However, they are associated with numerous urinary symptoms such as ureteric injuries, flank pain, etc. (Ramachandra et al. 2020; Rassweiler et al. 2017). Patients must retain the stent in situ for 4–6 weeks because conventional urethral stents necessitate cystoscopic extraction by a urologist, which is constrained by waiting times and availability of cystoscopy appointments in Hong Kong. The new magnetic double-J stents allow removal in a day ward setting, which can be performed by a urology nurse (Li et al. 2023; Ozturk 2017). As a result, a nurse-led double-J stent removal service was set up in August 2018 to provide early stent removal for these patients in Hong Kong.

Study Sharing: IV

A study recruited 60 patients between January 2019 and September 2019, with 30 having magnetic double-J stents and 30 having conventional double-J stents. There was no significant difference in median age between the groups (55.3 years for magnetic stents vs. 58.2 years for conventional stents, $P > 0.05$). However, the magnetic stent group had a significantly shorter median waiting time for stent removal (8 days vs. 35 days, $P < 0.05$) and removal time (2 min vs. 6 minutes, $P < 0.05$). The magnetic stent group also had significantly lower median pain score during removal (3.3 vs. 4.4 on visual analogue scale, $P < 0.05$) and lower International Prostate Symptom Score after removal (3.2 vs. 8.7, $P < 0.05$). In conclusion, magnetic double-J stents allowed faster removal with less pain compared to conventional stents.

Our early experience with magnetic double-J stents demonstrated that the device was convenient and well-tolerated by patients. The technique for stent removal is easily performed by urology nurses and applicable in nurse-led clinics. Furthermore, patients can benefit from early stent removal, which reduces stent-associated urinary symptoms.

The Impact of Virtual Reality on Pain, Anxiety, and Satisfaction During Transperineal Targeted and Systemic Prostate Biopsies

Due to the increasing prevalence of antibiotic-resistant bacteria and infectious complications associated with transrectal prostate biopsy, the TP approach is gaining wider adoption (Ortner et al. 2021; Wilcox et al. 2023). Given the invasive nature of the prostate biopsy procedure, there is potential for psychological trauma in patients regardless of the approach utilized. Patients undergoing TP prostate biopsies self-report moderate pain levels, and pre-procedural anxiety is predictive of increased pain perception (Huang et al. 2019; Udeh et al. 2015; Wilcox et al. 2023). Although medical hypnosis using virtual reality (VR) has demonstrated efficacy in reducing pain and anxiety during medical procedures, its potential in improving the patient experience during TP prostate biopsy has yet to be explored (Boyce et al. 2024; Candela et al. 2023; Genç et al. 2022; Vanoli et al. 2024). The following study aimed to investigate the effects of VR immersion on perceived anxiety and pain levels in patients undergoing TP prostate biopsy. Patients were recruited for this study between April 2022 and March 2023.

Study Sharing: V

This study investigated the effects of a VR intervention (HypnoVR) on patient-reported outcomes during TP prostate biopsy (Fig. 8.4). Sixty-four male patients undergoing TP biopsy by a single surgeon were non-randomly allocated to receive standard care (control group, $n = 28$) or standard care plus HypnoVR (experimental

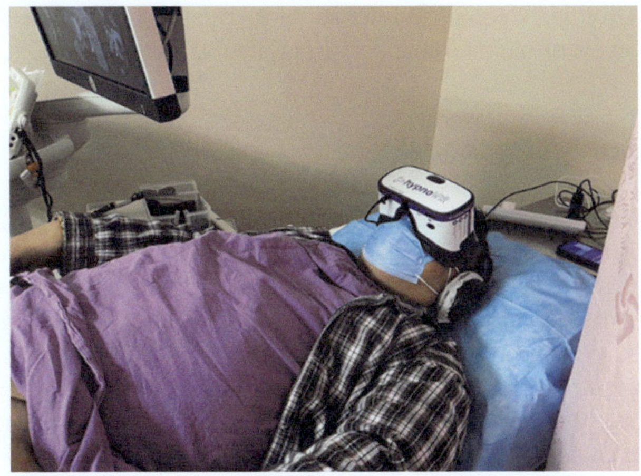

Fig. 8.4 Patient undergoing transperineal prostate biopsy while wearing the HypnoVR device, comprising a virtual reality headset and headphone

group, $n = 36$). All patients received a local anesthetic with 1% lidocaine per protocol. Using validated scales, patients self-reported pain tolerance, anxiety, and satisfaction immediately post-biopsy. There were no significant demographic or procedural differences between groups. The HypnoVR group reported significantly lower mean pain scores than the control group (4.19 vs. 5.25, $P < 0.05$). Among patients aged <65 years, HypnoVR resulted in significantly higher mean satisfaction scores (9 vs. 7.61, $P < 0.05$). Clinically meaningful reductions in pain, anxiety, and dissatisfaction were observed with HypnoVR during targeted TP biopsy specifically. No adverse events occurred. In conclusion, this initial study indicates HypnoVR may reduce self-reported pain and discomfort during TP prostate biopsy versus standard care alone. HypnoVR could provide a simple, cost-effective adjunct to sedation. Further rigorous evaluation in randomized controlled trials is warranted to substantiate these preliminary findings.

Developing and Validating a Visual Hematuria Grading Scale to Optimize Outcomes of Continuous Bladder Irrigation After Transurethral Resection of the Prostate

Hematuria is a common presenting symptom or secondary symptom for which patients seek medical evaluation and treatment by urology professionals (Bolenz et al. 2018). Nevertheless, thus far, no adequate tool for evaluating gross hematuria has emerged. The lack of a standardized assessment instrument creates uncertainty among healthcare professionals and patients when attempting to accurately convey the extent of gross hematuria (Madaan et al. 2021; Saleem and Hamawy 2022; Stout et al. 2021). Stout et al. (2021) developed and validated a hematuria grading scale that categorized 5 levels of hematuria with recommended actions for adjusting continuous bladder irrigation (CBI). The scale was designed for patients undergoing transurethral resection of the prostate (TURP) who receive CBI postoperatively.

Urologists conducted the study to create and validate the scale based on different levels of hematuria and appropriate CBI adjustments.

Study Sharing: VI

In a study conducted from October 2021 to March 2022, researchers examined 93 patients who suffered TURP. Forty-eight patients were managed postoperatively using a hematuria grading scale to guide CBI, while 45 patients did not use the scale. There was no significant difference between the groups in age, prostate size, surgery time, or amount of prostate resected. Patients using the hematuria scale required less CBI fluid (13.8 L vs. 38.4 L, $P < 0.05$) and shorter CBI duration (4.2 h vs. 11.9 h, $P < 0.05$) compared to those not using the scale. Clot retention needed manual irrigation occurred in 3 of 48 patients with the scale and 3 of 45 patients without ($P > 0.05$). Length of hospital stay was shorter with the hematuria scale (1.8 days vs. 2.5 days, $P < 0.05$). A nursing survey showed 90% satisfaction with using the hematuria scale to manage CBI.

This study evaluating the gross hematuria grading scale found high inter-rater reliability among healthcare providers across disciplines. The participating staff found the scale uncomplicated and practical to use. Implementation of a standardized hematuria grading method could prove beneficial for the evaluation and communication of gross hematuria presentations.

Conclusion

This chapter highlights new methods and practices in urology nursing care, concentrating on progressions and developments that add to enhanced patient results. The examinations led by Hong Kong urology nurses show the adequacy of different interventions in managing urological conditions and augmenting quality of life.

The use of new techniques, including hematuria scale, magnetic double-J stents, PTNS therapy, digital video for teaching catheter insertion, VR during prostate biopsies, and ESWT for ED, has shown good results. The hematuria scale was reliable and valid. Magnetic stents improve symptoms and quality of life. PTNS was a minimally invasive therapy for OAB. The video aided catheter insertion and confidence with self-catheterization. VR made biopsies safer and more comfortable. Shock wave therapy effectively treated ED. These innovations demonstrate potential for better outcomes in urology patients.

These findings contribute to ongoing efforts to improve urology care and provide evidence-based information for healthcare professionals worldwide. Urology nurse specialists play an important role in caring for urology patients by offering creative solutions and patient-centered care. As the shortage of urologists continues and the population ages, the role of urology nurses becomes more and more vital in ensuring quality urologic care and increasing patient satisfaction.

In conclusion, this chapter serves as a guidepost, illuminating the potential for urology nurse specialists to deliver high-quality, cost-effective care across diverse specialized areas of urological health. It emphasizes the significance of continuous learning and skill enhancement from an advanced practice perspective. Through the adoption of innovative approaches and techniques, urology nurse specialists can further augment their ability to provide individualized and efficacious care to urology patients.

References

Adeldaeim HM, Abouyoussif T, El Gebaly O, Assem A, Wahab MMA, Rashad H, Sakr M, Zahran AR (2021) Prognostic indicators for successful low-intensity extracorporeal shock wave therapy treatment of erectile dysfunction. Urology 149:133–139. https://doi.org/10.1016/j.urology.2020.12.019

Argiolas A, Argiolas FM, Argiolas G, Melis MR (2023) Erectile dysfunction: treatments, advances and new therapeutic strategies. Brain Sci 13(5):802. https://doi.org/10.3390/brainsci13050802

Atallah S, Haydar A, Jabbour T, Kfoury P, Sader G (2021) The effectiveness of psychological interventions alone, or in combination with phosphodiesterase-5 inhibitors, for the treatment of erectile dysfunction: a systematic review. Arab J Urol 19(3):310–322. https://doi.org/10.1080/2090598X.2021.1926763

Bocchino AC, Pezzoli M, Martínez-Salamanca JI, Russo GI, Giudice AL, Cocci A (2023) Low-intensity extracorporeal shock wave therapy for erectile dysfunction: myths and realities. Invest Clin Urol 64(2):118. https://doi.org/10.4111/icu.20220327

Bolenz C, Schröppel B, Eisenhardt A, Schmitz-Dräger BJ, Grimm MO (2018) The investigation of haematuria. Dtsch Arztebl Int 115(48):801. https://doi.org/10.3238/arztebl.2018.0801

Boyce L, Jordan C, Egan T, Sivaprakasam R (2024) Can virtual reality enhance the patient experience during awake invasive procedures? A systematic review of randomized controlled trials. Pain 165(4):741–752. https://doi.org/10.1097/j.pain.0000000000003086

Candela L, Ventimiglia E, Corrales M, Del Rio AS, Villa L, Goumas IK, Salonia A, Montorsi F, Doizi S, Traxer O (2023) The use of a virtual reality device (HypnoVR) during extracorporeal shockwave lithotripsy for treatment of urinary stones: initial results of a clinical protocol. Urology 175:13–17. https://doi.org/10.1016/j.urology.2023.01.048

Clavijo RI, Kohn TP, Kohn JR, Ramasamy R (2017) Effects of low-intensity extracorporeal shockwave therapy on erectile dysfunction: a systematic review and meta-analysis. J Sex Med 14(1):27–35. https://doi.org/10.1016/j.jsxm.2016.11.001

Corcos J, Przydacz M, Campeau L, Witten J, Hickling D, Honeine C, Radomski SB, Stothers L, Wagg A (2017) CUA guideline on adult overactive bladder. Can Urol Assoc J 11(5):E142. https://doi.org/10.5489/cuaj.4586

Li J, Gauhar V, Lim EJ, Dmitriy S, Vladimir O, Dmitriy G, Igor S, Gadzhiev N (2023) Safety and effectiveness of magnetic ureteric stent removal under ultrasound control: a randomized single center trial. World J Urol 41(11):2889–2896. https://doi.org/10.1007/s00345-023-04437-5

Genç H, Korkmaz M, Akkurt A (2022) The effect of virtual reality glasses and stress balls on pain and vital findings during transrectal prostate biopsy: a randomized controlled trial. J Perianesth Nurs 37(3):344–350. https://doi.org/10.1016/j.jopan.2021.09.006

Huang GL, Kang CH, Lee WC, Chiang PH (2019) Comparisons of cancer detection rate and complications between transrectal and transperineal prostate biopsy approaches – a single center preliminary study. BMC Urol 19:1–8. https://doi.org/10.1186/s12894-019-0539-4

Hentzen C, Haddad R, Ismael SS, Peyronnet B, Gamé X, Denys P, Robain G, Amarenco G, Manceau P (2019) Predictive factors of adherence to urinary self-catheterization in older adults. Neurourol Urodyn 38(2):770–778. https://doi.org/10.1002/nau.23915

Lajiness M, Quallich S (2016) The nurse practitioner in urology, vol 198. Springer

Lawler AC, Ghiraldi EM, Tong C, Friedlander JI (2017) Extracorporeal shock wave therapy: current perspectives and future directions. Curr Urol Rep 18:1–7. https://doi.org/10.1007/s11934-017-0672-0

Lu Z, Lin G, Reed-Maldonado A, Wang C, Lee YC, Lue TF (2017) Low-intensity extracorporeal shock wave treatment improves erectile function: a systematic review and meta-analysis. Eur Urol 71(2):223–233. https://doi.org/10.1016/j.eururo.2016.05.050

Man L, Li G (2018) Low-intensity extracorporeal shock wave therapy for erectile dysfunction: a systematic review and meta-analysis. Urology 119:97–103. https://doi.org/10.1016/j.urology.2017.09.011

Madaan A, Kuusk T, Hamdoon M, Elliott A, Pearce D, Madaan S (2021) Nurse-led one stop haematuria clinic: outcomes from 2,714 patients. BJUI Compass 2(6):385–394. https://doi.org/10.1002/bco2.100

Madeira CR, Tonin FS, Fachi MM, Borba HH, Ferreira VL, Leonart LP, Bonetti AF, Moritz RP, Trindade ACLB, Gonçalves AG, Fernandez-Llimos F, Pontarolo R (2021) Efficacy and safety of oral phosphodiesterase 5 inhibitors for erectile dysfunction: a network meta-analysis and multicriteria decision analysis. World J Urol 39:953–962. https://doi.org/10.1007/s00345-020-03233-9

Newman DK, Rovner ES, Wein AJ, Goetz LL, Droste L, Klausner AP, Newman DK (2018) Catheters used for intermittent catheterization. In: Clinical application of urologic catheters, devices and products. Springer, Cham, pp 47–77

Ortner G, Tzanaki E, Rai BP, Nagele U, Tokas T (2021) Transperineal prostate biopsy: the modern gold standard to prostate cancer diagnosis. Turk J Urol 47(Suppl 1):S19. https://doi.org/10.5152/tud.2020.20358

Ozturk H (2017) Facilitate stent removal: magnetic DJ stent. Urol Case Rep 11:5. https://doi.org/10.1016/j.eucr.2016.11.021

Peters KM, Carrico DJ, Perez-Marrero RA, Khan AU, Wooldridge LS, Davis GL, MacDiarmid SA (2010) Randomized trial of percutaneous tibial nerve stimulation versus Sham efficacy in the treatment of overactive bladder syndrome: results from the SUmiT trial. J Urol 183(4):1438–1443. https://doi.org/10.1016/j.juro.2009.12.036

Quallich, S. A., & Lajiness, M. J. (Eds.). (2020). The nurse practitioner in urology: a manual for nurse practitioners, physician assistants and allied healthcare providers. Springer Nature

Ramachandra M, Mosayyebi A, Carugo D, Somani BK (2020) Strategies to improve patient outcomes and QOL: current complications of the design and placements of ureteric stents. Res Rep Urol 12:303–314. https://doi.org/10.2147/RRU.S233981

Ramírez-García I, Blanco-Ratto L, Kauffmann S, Carralero-Martínez A, Sánchez E (2019) Efficacy of transcutaneous stimulation of the posterior tibial nerve compared to percutaneous stimulation in idiopathic overactive bladder syndrome: randomized control trial. Neurourol Urodyn 38(1):261–268. https://doi.org/10.1002/nau.23843

Rassweiler MC, Michel MS, Ritter M, Honeck P (2017) Magnetic ureteral stent removal without cystoscopy: a randomized controlled trial. J Endourol 31(8):762–766. https://doi.org/10.1089/end.2017.0051

Rola, P., Włodarczak, A., Barycki, M., & Doroszko, A. (2022). Use of the shock wave therapy in basic research and clinical applications—from bench to bedsite. Biomedicine, 10(3), 568. https://doi.org/10.3390/biomedicines10030568

Saleem MO, Hamawy K. (2022) Haematuria. In: StatPearls [Internet]. StatPearls Publishing. Available: https://www.ncbi.nlm.nih.gov/books/NBK534213/

Scarneciu I, Lupu S, Bratu OG, Teodorescu A, Maxim LS, Brinza A, Laculiceanu AG, Rotaru RM, Lupu A, Scarneciu CC (2021) Overactive bladder: a review and update. Exp Ther Med 22(6):1–8. https://doi.org/10.3892/etm.2021.10879

Stout TE, Borofsky M, Soubra A (2021) A visual scale for improving communication when describing gross haematuria. Urology 148:32–36. https://doi.org/10.1016/j.urology.2020.10.054

Udeh, E. I., Amu, O. C., Nnabugwu, I. I., & Ozoemena, O. F. N. (2015). Transperineal versus transrectal prostate biopsy: our findings in a tertiary health institution. Niger J Clin Pract, 18(1), 110–114. https://doi.org/10.4103/1119-3077.146991

Vanoli S, Grobet-Jeandin E, Windisch O, Valerio M, Benamran D (2024) Evolution of anxiety management in prostate biopsy under local anesthesia: a narrative review. World J Urol 42(1):43. https://doi.org/10.1007/s00345-023-04723-2

Wang X, Cao X, Li J, Deng C, Wang T, Fu L, Zhang Q (2021) Evaluation of patient-reported outcome measures in intermittent self-catheterization users: a systematic review. Arch Phys Med Rehabil 102(11):2239–2246. https://doi.org/10.1016/j.apmr.2021.03.020

Wilcox VB, George AK, Kaye DR (2023) Should transperineal prostate biopsy be the standard of care? Curr Urol Rep 24(3):135–142. https://doi.org/10.1007/s11934-022-01139-0

Yafi FA, Jenkins L, Albersen M, Corona G, Isidori AM, Goldfarb S, Maggi M, Nelson CJ, Parish S, Salonia A, Tan R, Mulhall JP, Hellstrom WJ (2016) Erectile dysfunction. Nat Rev Dis Primers 2(1):1–20. https://doi.org/10.1038/nrdp.2016.3

Part III

Care Needs and Transitions

Bridging Communication and Culture: Advanced Nursing Strategies for Colorectal Cancer Care in Chinese Communities

Choi-Ping Lam, Alice Yip, and Jeff Yip

Introduction

In the bustling corridors of Hong Kong's hospitals, a quiet revolution is taking place. Traditional Chinese beliefs about cancer—where the word itself whispers of inevitable death—are being challenged by specialized nurses who understand that healing extends far beyond medical treatment. In many cultures, particularly within traditional Chinese society, "cancer" often evokes profound dread, associated with incurability and death. This perception, rooted in historical beliefs and cultural narratives, frequently leads to families shielding patients from the full truth, thereby reinforcing cancer as an insurmountable foe (Pergolizzi et al. 2024).

However, the World Health Organization (WHO) now recognizes cancer as a chronic disease, akin to other long-term conditions like diabetes or heart disease (WHO 2025). This reclassification necessitates a paradigm shift in how cancer is communicated, perceived, and managed, especially in cultural contexts where fear and stigma have historically dominated.

Colorectal nurses, through their continuous presence and holistic approach, are uniquely positioned at the forefront of this evolving healthcare landscape. They serve as crucial bridges, translating complex medical advancements into understandable terms while honoring cultural values and family dynamics. Advanced

C.-P. Lam
Prince of Wales Hospital, Shatin, HKSAR, China
e-mail: lcp660@ha.org.hk

A. Yip (✉)
School of Health Sciences, St. Francis University,
Tseung Kwan O, Hong Kong
e-mail: khyip@sfu.edu.hk

J. Yip
Tung Wah College, Ho Man Tin, HKSAR, China
e-mail: jeffreyyip@twc.edu.hk

A. Yip, G. D. Smith (eds.), *Surgical Nursing in Practice*,
https://doi.org/10.1007/978-3-032-14729-5_9

nursing skills, with empathetic and culturally sensitive approaches, profoundly influence patient outcomes and the journey from diagnosis to survivorship in Hong Kong's unique healthcare context.

Understanding Colorectal Cancer in Hong Kong's Context

Colorectal cancer (CRC) represents more than statistics in Hong Kong—it affects families, communities, and cultural traditions. In 2022, CRC was the third most common malignancy in Hong Kong, with 5190 new cases recorded. This significant incidence rate emphasizes the increasingly vital role of specialized nursing care in managing the disease and supporting patients (Hong Kong Cancer Registry 2024). CRC was also the third leading cause of cancer-related deaths in the same year, responsible for 14.7% of all new cancer cases (Centre for Health Protection 2025).

Treatment options encompass surgery, chemotherapy, radiation therapy, targeted therapy, and immunotherapy (Kumar et al. 2023). Surgery remains the cornerstone of curative treatment, particularly for early-stage disease (Eng et al. 2022). For locally advanced rectal cancer, neoadjuvant chemotherapy and radiation therapy may precede surgery to optimize outcomes. These decisions emerge from multidisciplinary team discussions involving surgeons, oncologists, radiologists, and critically, colorectal nurses.

Within this collaborative framework, colorectal nurses translate complex medical information into culturally appropriate language, integrate patient values with clinical recommendations, coordinate care transitions, and advocate for holistic approaches that prioritize both medical outcomes and quality of life (Colomer-Lahiguera et al. 2024).

Advanced Nursing Competency in Breaking Bad News: The SPIKES Protocol

The art of delivering difficult news requires cultural sensitivity, emotional intelligence, and refined communication skills (Yip et al. 2021). As colorectal nurses, we have developed expertise in delivering sensitive information through the SPIKES protocol—encompassing Setting, Perception, Invitation, Knowledge, Empathy, and Strategy & Summary—adapted for Chinese families in Hong Kong (Baile et al. 2000).

Cultural Context: Navigating Traditional Chinese Approaches

Traditional Chinese culture often emphasizes family protection through information control, particularly regarding serious illnesses affecting elderly family members. This practice, rooted in filial piety, stems from the belief that cancer diagnoses may cause overwhelming distress (Lewandowska et al. 2021). Family members frequently request that diagnoses be withheld, creating ethical dilemmas for healthcare providers.

Advanced practice colorectal nurses acknowledge that certain well-intentioned cultural practices cause anxiety and impede informed decision-making. Their role requires navigating these complexities while advocating for patient autonomy and fostering trust-based therapeutic relationships (Cranstoun et al. 2024).

Perception (P): Understanding the Patient's Inner World

Research consistently demonstrates that patients across cultures desire health information. A landmark 1982 survey of 1251 Americans revealed that 96% wished to be informed of a cancer diagnosis, while 85% wanted realistic prognostic information (Cassileth et al. 1980). Similarly, European studies showed that 91% and 94% of patients wanted to know their chances of cure and potential treatment side effects, respectively (Meredith et al. 1996).

Patients often perceive the gravity of their condition prior to diagnosis. When this perception is unacknowledged by clinicians, it can heighten frustration, anxiety, and isolation. Assessment, therefore, requires observing verbal and nonverbal cues, exploring understanding, and creating a safe environment for inquiry (Crivelli et al. 2024).

Invitation (I): Respecting the Pace of Understanding

The "Invitation" component represents crucial respect for patient autonomy and Readiness (Mahendiran et al. 2023; von Blanckenburg et al. 2020). This step involves explicitly asking patients for permission to share information, acknowledging that timing and extent of disclosure should align with their emotional preparedness.

When patients indicate they are not ready for detailed discussions, we respect this choice while ensuring they understand that information will be available when they feel prepared (Yip et al. 2021). This approach empowers patients to control their learning journey while maintaining open communication channels.

Knowledge (K): The Art of Compassionate Truth-Telling

Delivering difficult medical information requires skill in translating complex concepts into understandable, culturally appropriate language (Mahendiran et al. 2023; von Blanckenburg et al. 2020). Effective knowledge sharing avoids medical jargon while maintaining accuracy and hope. Rather than delivering blunt statements, we use graduated disclosure that allows patients to process information incrementally.

This approach respects the Chinese cultural preference for indirect communication while ensuring patients receive essential information for informed decision-making (Pun et al. 2020).

Case Study: Transforming Fear into Agency

This case study examines the critical role of culturally sensitive communication in colorectal nursing. The patient, an 80-year-old woman diagnosed with locally advanced rectal cancer, initially presented with a family-imposed narrative of a benign *large polyp*. This protective deception, rooted in cultural values, created a barrier to informed consent and caused the patient significant distress as her symptoms worsened.

The turning point occurred during a family meeting facilitated by the colorectal nurse. Recognizing the patient's suspicion and the family's intent to shield her from harm, the colorectal nurse mediated a dialogue. This intervention focused on explaining that the patient's awareness of her deteriorating condition was already causing emotional harm and that her participation was vital for effective treatment.

Applying principles like the SPIKES protocol, which provides a framework for delivering difficult news, the colorectal nurse first addressed the patient's own perceptions. Acknowledging the seriousness of her condition validated her experience and fostered trust. The subsequent disclosure of the diagnosis was met not with despair but with empowered resolve. The patient's question, "what do we need to do?" signaled a shift from a state of isolated confusion to one of agency and collaboration.

This case demonstrates that direct, empathic communication, when delivered with cultural humility, does not necessarily cause the harm families may fear. Instead, it can empower patients, respect their autonomy, and unify families in developing a therapeutic plan. The colorectal nurse's intervention transformed the care dynamic, emphasis that truth, skilfully and compassionately delivered, is foundational to patient-centered care.

Psychosocial Dimensions of Colorectal Cancer Care

The psychological and social impact of colorectal cancer extends far beyond physical symptoms, particularly within Chinese cultural contexts, where communication patterns, family dynamics, and social expectations create unique challenges (Li et al. 2018; Yoon et al. 2020).

Breaking the Silence: Understanding Male Patients' Communication Patterns

Chinese cultural values often emphasize emotional restraint, particularly among men, who may view silence as a virtue (Khoo et al. 2022; Yuan et al. 2025). This cultural stoicism can significantly impact cancer care, as male patients may delay reporting symptoms, minimize emotional distress, or avoid seeking support even from their spouses.

Male colorectal cancer patients often attempt to shield their families from worry by maintaining a facade of strength. While this stems from love and protective instincts, it often creates situations where incomplete information increases family anxiety and impedes effective support.

Confronting Stigma and Emotional Responses

Cancer diagnosis triggers intense emotional responses, including fear, anxiety, and depression. Within Chinese cultural contexts, these may be complicated by beliefs linking illness to personal failings or karmic consequences (Song et al. 2020; Wang et al. 2022). Colorectal cancer presents additional challenges related to body image and dignity, particularly when treatment involves stoma creation (Khoo et al. 2022).

Nursing practice addresses these concerns by incorporating comprehensive psychosocial assessment, validating emotional responses, providing education on cancer causation, and connecting patients with culturally appropriate support resources.

Survivorship and Fear of Recurrence

The transition from active treatment to survivorship brings unique psychological challenges, with *Fear of Cancer Recurrence* (FCR), representing one of the most significant concerns (Nahm et al. 2021; Yip et al. 2021). This fear manifests as intrusive thoughts about cancer returning and anxiety about the future, particularly pronounced during the first 3 years following treatment (Luigjes-Huizer et al. 2022).

Effective Communication Strategies and Shared Decision-Making

Advanced communication skills form the cornerstone of effective colorectal nursing practice, particularly when working with Chinese families, where decision-making often involves multiple generations and complex cultural considerations.

Transforming Fear into Understanding: Addressing Stoma-Related Anxiety

The prospect of stoma creation is a significant source of anxiety for colorectal cancer patients, frequently stemming from misconceptions about stoma function and a feared loss of dignity (Tan et al. 2024; Xue et al. 2025). These anxieties can be magnified within cultural frameworks, such as Chinese culture, that place deep significance on bodily wholeness and social harmony (Khoo et al. 2022).

A therapeutic nursing approach seeks to transform this fear into understanding and agency (Hu et al. 2025; Harris et al. 2020; Yip et al. 2021). The intervention begins by validating patient concerns while systematically providing accurate, hope-filled information. Preoperative, hands-on education with modern stoma products helps to illustrate daily management, such as odor-control features, and secure adhesion systems, demonstrating that contemporary appliances are both effective and discreet (Harris et al. 2020; Yeo and Park 2023). This counseling includes detailed discussions about surgical procedures and practical concerns such as pain management, dietary modifications, and lifestyle adaptations; addresses practical recovery aspects; and navigates culturally specific challenges related to family roles and social participation (family gatherings, traditional festivals).

A critical component of this process is connection patients with peer support networks, such as the Hong Kong Stoma Association. Narratives from volunteers with shared cultural backgrounds are particularly potent. They normalize experience, reduce feelings of isolation, and provide tangible proof that a fulfilling life—including meaningful relationships, careers, and social activities—remains entirely achievable post-surgery. This multifaceted strategy empowers patients to move beyond fear toward informed acceptance and active participation in their care.

Facilitating Informed Decision-Making

Facilitating informed colorectal cancer decisions requires synthesizing complex treatment data with patient values and cultural contexts (Petersén and Carlsson 2021). We translate clinical information, considering cancer stages and health, to align treatment plans with patient-centered quality of life priorities, ensuring a truly personalized approach to care (Goldenberg et al. 2020; Lin et al. 2024).

Multidisciplinary Collaboration and Nursing Leadership

The multidisciplinary team approach represents the gold standard for colorectal cancer management (National Comprehensive Cancer Network 2024). Within this framework, colorectal nurses provide unique contributions by presenting the holistic patient picture, including psychosocial factors, family dynamics, and cultural considerations.

Nurturing Survivorship: Beyond Treatment Completion

The transition from active treatment to survivorship represents a critical phase requiring specialized nursing support (Simard et al. 2019). This period presents unique opportunities for health promotion and long-term well-being (Tabriz et al. 2023).

Understanding the Survivorship Transition

The survivorship transition is often marked by heightened health consciousness that declines posttreatment (Luo et al. 2021). Nursing interventions must therefore emphasize the chronicity of cancer care and the critical need to adopt sustainable lifestyle modifications for long-term well-being.

Comprehensive Fear of Recurrence Management

Fear of cancer recurrence is a prevalent issue for a majority of cancer survivors, characterized by ongoing worry and heightened awareness of physical symptoms (Luigjes-Huizer et al. 2022; Zhang et al. 2022). A comprehensive management approach involves normalizing these fears while equipping patients with practical strategies to manage anxiety (Lim et al. 2025). Among these strategies, regular exercise stands out as a powerful intervention (Oruç and Kaplan 2019). There is strong evidence that structured physical activity not only aids in managing anxiety and depression but also significantly reduces the risk of colorectal cancer recurrence (Ho et al. 2020; Oruç and Kaplan 2019; Singh et al. 2020).

Culturally Sensitive Lifestyle Education

Our survivorship approach integrates evidence-based guidelines with Chinese cultural values and practical constraints to promote holistic health and well-being (Luo et al. 2021; Mao et al. 2022; Wong et al. 2021).

Nutrition counseling matches evidence-based guidelines with traditional Chinese nutritious practices. Emphasis is placed on culturally familiar, high-fiber foods and adapting recipes to enhance nutritional content while preserving palatability. Guidance on portion control, meal timing, and integrating nutrient-dense foods facilitates adherence within established dietary patterns.

Physical activity recommendations emphasize accessible, culturally congruent exercises, like Tai Chi and Qigong. Goal setting is progressive and individualized, respecting patient limitations and sociocultural contexts. These traditional modalities offer comparable efficacy to Western fitness programs in promoting long-term health and cancer prevention, ensuring sustainable engagement for patients.

Weight management guidance promotes maintaining a healthy body mass index to reduce recurrence risk while respecting cultural attitudes toward body image. Practical strategies, including portion control and mindful eating, are adapted to sociocultural contexts, like communal meals to ensure cultural relevance and adherence.

Culturally tailored cessation support addresses sociocultural barriers, such as social smoking and traditional beliefs. The critical importance of quitting for cancer survivors is emphasized, with practical, evidence-based strategies provided to overcome addiction and prevent relapse.

Stress management integrates modern techniques, such as mindfulness, with traditional Chinese practices like meditation and gentle movement. This facilitates personalized coping strategies that align with individual lifestyles, stress triggers, and cultural preferences.

Surveillance education promotes adherence to follow-up schedules and symptom recognition while mitigating anxiety over benign sensations. Clear, bilingual written materials are provided to patients and families, ensuring information is accessible and comprehensible in their preferred language.

Building Comprehensive Support Systems

Effective colorectal cancer care encompasses comprehensive support systems addressing the needs of patients, families, and caregivers throughout the cancer journey.

Institutional and Community Resources

Hong Kong's healthcare system provides multiple support layers including hospital-based services and community organizations, such as the Hong Kong Cancer Fund and Hong Kong Anti-Cancer Society. We facilitate connections between patients and these resources, recognizing that different patients benefit from different types of support.

Peer Support and Family Care

Peer support offers an invaluable resource through survivor-led groups. Recognizing the familial impact, comprehensive caregiver support, including educational, emotional, and stress management resources, is also provided to address the needs of the entire family unit.

Conclusion

The role of colorectal nurses in Hong Kong transforms traditional clinical duties, encompassing cultural contribution, patient advocacy, and health promotion. By integrating advanced communication skills and cultural competence, these nurses enhance cancer care in multicultural settings. The culturally adapted SPIKES protocol, for instance, provides a strong framework for delivering difficult news while respecting family dynamics and patient autonomy.

Psychosocial care requires attention to cultural factors that influence communication and help-seeking behaviors. Furthermore, survivorship care is an emerging specialty focused on long-term effects and health promotion.

As healthcare moves toward patient-centered models, the ability of colorectal nurses to navigate complex cultural dynamics while providing evidence-based care positions them as indispensable leaders. Their work reveals a future where cancer is not only medically excellent but also culturally responsive and profoundly humane.

References

Baile WF, Buckman R, Lenzi R, Glober G, Beale EA, Kudelka AP (2000) SPIKES—a six-step protocol for delivering bad news: application to the patient with cancer. Oncologist 5(4):302–311. https://doi.org/10.1634/theonocologist.5-4-302

Cassileth BR, Zupkis RV, Sutton-Smith K, March V (1980) Information and participation preferences among cancer patients. Ann Intern Med 92(6):832–836. https://doi.org/10.7326/0003-4819-92-6-832

Centre for Health Protection (2025) Colorectal cancer. Department of Health the Government of the Hong Kong Special Administrative Region. Online available: https://www.chp.gov.hk/en/healthtopics/content/25/51.html. Accessed on 30 July 2025

Colomer-Lahiguera S, Gentizon J, Christofis M, Darnac C, Serena A, Eicher M (2024) Achieving comprehensive, patient-centered cancer services: optimizing the role of advanced practice nurses at the core of precision health. Semin Oncol Nurs 40(3):151629. https://doi.org/10.1016/j.soncn.2024.151629

Cranstoun D, Baliousis M, Merdian HL, Rennoldson M (2024) Nurse-led psychological interventions for depression in adult cancer patients: a systematic review and meta-analysis of randomized controlled trials. J Pain Symptom Manag 68(1):e21–e35. https://doi.org/10.1016/j.jpainsymman.2024.03.028

Crivelli AF, Barello S, Acampora M, Bonetti L (2024) Uncovering nursing communication strategies and relational styles to foster patient engagement in oncology: a scoping review. Healthcare 12(13):1261. https://doi.org/10.3390/healthcare12131261

Eng C, Jacome AA, Agarwal R, Hayat MH, Byndloss MX, Holowatyj AN, Bailey C, Lieu CH (2022) A comprehensive framework for early-onset colorectal cancer research. Lancet Oncol 23(3):e116–e128. https://doi.org/10.1016/S1470-2045(21)00588-X

Goldenberg BA, Carpenter-Kellett T, Gingerich JR, Nugent Z, Sisler JJ (2020) Moving forward after cancer: successful implementation of a colorectal cancer patient–centered transitions program. J Cancer Surviv 14(1):4–8. https://doi.org/10.1007/s11764-019-00819-0

Harris MS, Kelly K, Paris C (2020) Does preoperative ostomy education decrease anxiety in the new ostomy patient? A quantitative comparison cohort study. J Wound Ostomy Continence Nurs 47(2):137–139. https://doi.org/10.1097/WON.000000000000062

Ho M, Ho JW, Fong DY, Lee CF, Macfarlane DJ, Cerin E, Lee AM, Leung S, Chan WYY, Leung IPF, Lam SHS, Chu N, Taylor AJ, Cheng KK (2020) Effects of dietary and physical activity interventions on generic and cancer-specific health-related quality of life, anxiety, and depression in colorectal cancer survivors: a randomized controlled trial. J Cancer Surviv 14(4):424–433. https://doi.org/10.1007/s11764-020-00864-0

Hong Kong Cancer Registry (2024) Overview of Hong Kong cancer statistics of 2022. Hong Kong Hospital Authority. Online available: https://www3.ha.org.hk/cancereg. Accessed on 30 July 2025

Hu M, Tingting A, Zhang X, Huang X, Wu Q, Wei T, Song B, Hu S (2025) Attitudes toward seeking professional psychological help among patients with colorectal cancer: a latent profile analysis. Asia Pac J Oncol Nurs:100755. https://doi.org/10.1016/j.apjon.2025.100755

Khoo AMG, Lau J, Loh XS, Ng CWT, Griva K, Tan KK (2022) Understanding the psychosocial impact of colorectal cancer on young-onset patients: a scoping review. Cancer Med 11(7):1688–1700. https://doi.org/10.1002/cam4.4575

Kumar A, Gautam V, Sandhu A, Rawat K, Sharma A, Saha L (2023) Current and emerging therapeutic approaches for colorectal cancer: a comprehensive review. World J Gastrointest Surg 15(4):495. https://doi.org/10.4240/wjgs.v15.i4.495

Lewandowska A, Rudzki G, Lewandowski T, Rudzki S (2021) The problems and needs of patients diagnosed with cancer and their caregivers. Int J Environ Res Public Health 18(1):87. https://doi.org/10.3390/ijerph18010087

Li Q, Lin Y, Chen Y, Loke AY (2018) Mutual support and challenges among Chinese couples living with colorectal cancer: a qualitative study. Cancer Nurs 41(5):E50–E60. https://doi.org/10.1097/NCC.0000000000000553

Lim CYS, Laidsaar-Powell RC, Young JM, Solomon M, Steffens D, Blinman P, O'Loughlin S, Zhang Y, Butow P, advanced-CRC survivorship authorship group (2025) Fear of cancer progression and death anxiety in survivors of advanced colorectal cancer: a qualitative study exploring coping strategies and quality of life. Omega-J Death Dying 90(3):1325–1362. https://doi.org/10.1177/00302228221121493

Lin L, Fang Y, Wei Y, Huang F, Zheng J, Xiao H (2024) The effects of a nurse-led discharge planning on the health outcomes of colorectal cancer patients with stomas: a randomized controlled trial. Int J Nurs Stud 155:104769. https://doi.org/10.1016/j.ijnurstu.2024.104769

Luigjes-Huizer YL, Tauber NM, Humphris G, Kasparian NA, Lam WW, Lebel S, Simard S, Smith AB, Zachariae R, Afiyanti Y, Bell KJL, Custers JAE, de Wit NJ, Fisher PL, Galica J, Garland SN, Helsper CW, Jeppesen MM, Liu J, Mititelu R, Monninkhof EM, Russell L, Savard J, Speckens AEM, van Helmondt SJ, Vatandoust S, Zdenkowski N, van der Lee ML (2022) What is the prevalence of fear of cancer recurrence in cancer survivors and patients? A systematic review and individual participant data meta-analysis. Psycho-Oncology 31(6):879–892. https://doi.org/10.1002/pon.5921

Luo X, Li J, Chen M, Gong J, Xu Y, Li Q (2021) A literature review of post-treatment survivorship interventions for colorectal cancer survivors and/or their caregivers. Psycho-Oncology 30(6):807–817. https://doi.org/10.1002/pon.5657

Mahendiran M, Yeung H, Rossi S, Khosravani H, Perri GA (2023) Evaluating the effectiveness of the SPIKES model to break bad news–a systematic review. Am J Hosp Palliat Med 40(11):1231–1260. https://doi.org/10.1177/10499091221146296

Mao JJ, Pillai GG, Andrade CJ, Ligibel JA, Basu P, Cohen L, Khan IA, Mustian KM, Puthiyedath R, Dhiman KS, Lao L, Ghelman R, Guido PC, Lopez G, Gallego-Perez DF, Salicrup LA (2022) Integrative oncology: addressing the global challenges of cancer prevention and treatment. CA Cancer J Clin 72(2):144–164. https://doi.org/10.3322/caac.21706

Meredith C, Symonds P, Webster L, Lamont D, Pyper E, Gillis CR, Fallowfield L (1996) Information needs of cancer patients in West Scotland: cross sectional survey of patients' views. BMJ 313(7059):724–726. https://doi.org/10.1136/bmj.313.7059.724

Nahm SH, Blinman P, Butler S, Tan SC, Vardy J (2021) Factors associated with fear of cancer recurrence in breast and colorectal cancer survivors: a cross-sectional study of cancer survivors. Asia Pac J Clin Oncol 17(3):222–229. https://doi.org/10.1111/ajco.13434

National Comprehensive Cancer Network (2024) NCCN guidelines for patients: colon cancer. Online available: https://www.nccn.org/patients/guidelines/content/PDF/colon-patient.pdf

Oruç Z, Kaplan MA (2019) Effect of exercise on colorectal cancer prevention and treatment. World J Gastrointest Oncol 11(5):348. https://doi.org/10.4251/wjgo.v11.i5.348

Pergolizzi JJ, LeQuang JAK, Wagner M, Varrassi G (2024) Challenges in palliative care in Latin America: a narrative review. Cureus 16(5):e60698. https://doi.org/10.7759/cureus.60698

Petersén C, Carlsson E (2021) Life with a stoma—coping with daily life: experiences from focus group interviews. J Clin Nurs 30(15–16):2309–2319. https://doi.org/10.1111/jocn.15769

Pun JK, Cheung KM, Chow JC, Chan WL (2020) Chinese perspective on end-of-life communication: a systematic review. BMJ Support Palliat Care 14(e1):e30–e37. https://doi.org/10.1136/bmjspcare-2019-002166

Simard J, Kamath S, Kircher S (2019) Survivorship guidance for patients with colorectal cancer. Curr Treat Options in Oncol 20(5):38. https://doi.org/10.1007/s11864-019-0635-4

Singh B, Hayes SC, Spence RR, Steele ML, Millet GY, Gergele L (2020) Exercise and colorectal cancer: a systematic review and meta-analysis of exercise safety, feasibility and effectiveness. Int J Behav Nutr Phys Act 17(1):122. https://doi.org/10.1186/s12966-020-01021-7

Song L, Han X, Zhang J, Tang L (2020) Body image mediates the effect of stoma status on psychological distress and quality of life in patients with colorectal cancer. Psycho-Oncology 29(4):796–802. https://doi.org/10.1002/pon.5352

Tabriz ER, Ramezani M, Heydari A, Aledavood SA (2023) Health-promoting lifestyle among the survivors of colorectal cancer: an integrative review. J Caring Sci 12(3):201. https://doi.org/10.34172/jcs.2023.31768

Tan Z, Jiang L, Lu A, He X, Zuo Y, Yang J (2024) Living with a permanent ostomy: a descriptive phenomenological study on postsurgical experiences in patients with colorectal cancer. BMJ Open 14(11):e087959. https://doi.org/10.1136/bmjopen-2024-087959

von Blanckenburg P, Hofmann M, Rief W, Seifart U, Seifart C (2020) Assessing patients preferences for breaking bad news according to the SPIKES-protocol: the MABBAN scale. Patient Educ Couns 103(8):1623–1629. https://doi.org/10.1016/j.pec.2020.02.036

Wang Y, Li S, Gong J, Cao L, Xu D, Yu Q, Wang X, Chen Y (2022) Perceived stigma and self-efficacy of patients with inflammatory bowel disease-related stoma in China: a cross-sectional study. Front Med 9:813367. https://doi.org/10.3389/fmed.2022.813367

Wong JYH, Ho JWC, Lee AM, Fong DYT, Chu N, Leung S, Chan YYW, Lam SHS, Leung IPF, Macfarlane D, Cerin E, Taylor A, Cheng KK (2021) Lived experience of dietary change among Chinese colorectal cancer survivors in Hong Kong: a qualitative study. BMJ Open 11(8):e051052. https://doi.org/10.1136/bmjopen-2021-051052

World Health Organization (2025) Cancer. Online available: https://www.who.int/news-room/fact-sheets/detail/cancer

Xue Y, Lv K, Yuan C, Fan G, Yu P (2025) The experience and needs of self-care in elderly colorectal cancer stoma patients: a qualitative study. Support Care Cancer 33(6):474. https://doi.org/10.1007/s00520-025-09530-6

Yeo H, Park H (2023) Benefits of a single-session, in-hospital preoperative education program for patients undergoing ostomy surgery: a randomized controlled trial. J Wound Ostomy Cont Nurs 50(4):313–318. https://doi.org/10.1097/WON.0000000000000991

Yip YC, Tsui WK, Yip KH (2021) Hong Kong's growing need for palliative care services and the role of the nursing profession. Asia Pac J Health Manag 16(1)., i597:1–7. https://doi.org/10.24083/apjhm.v16i1.597

Yoon S, Chua TB, Tan IB, Matchar D, Ong MEH, Tan E (2020) Living with long-term consequences: experience of follow-up care and support needs among Asian long-term colorectal cancer survivors. Psycho-Oncology 29(10):1557–1563. https://doi.org/10.1002/pon.5452

Yuan C, Xie J, Cui L, Du Q, Li X, Wang X, Liu J, Wu X, Zhang M (2025) Psychosocial adjustment and influencing factors in patients with newly diagnosed colorectal cancer: a latent profile analysis. Eur J Oncol Nurs 75:102818. https://doi.org/10.1016/j.ejon.2025.102818

Zhang X, Sun D, Qin N, Liu M, Jiang N, Li X (2022) Factors correlated with fear of cancer recurrence in cancer survivors: a meta-analysis. Cancer Nurs 45(5):406–415. https://doi.org/10.1097/NCC.0000000000001020

Elevating Patient Outcomes: The Synergy of Advanced Nursing Practice and Compassionate Care in Breast Disease Management by Breast Care Nurses

10

Shuk-Yu Maria Hung, Kwai-Ying Wong, and Alice Yip

Introduction

Cancer is one of the leading causes of death worldwide. The most prevalent types of cancer include breast, lung, colon, rectal, and prostate cancers (World Health Organization 2025a). However, breast cancer is the most commonly diagnosed cancer among women worldwide (World Health Organization 2025b), including Hong Kong (Centre for Health Protection, HKSAR, 24 February 2025). It is the leading cause of cancer-related deaths in this population (International Agency for Research on Cancer, World Health Organization 2025). Over 2.3 million women were diagnosed with breast cancer, resulting in 670,000 deaths worldwide in 2022 (World Health Organization 2025b). It is forecasted that about 3.2 million new cases and over 1.1 million deaths will occur in 2050 (Devi 2025). It can affect women of any age after puberty worldwide, but the prevalence rises with age later in life. Early detection, combined with advanced surgical treatments and oncological interventions, is vital for improving survival rates. A diagnosis elicits fear, uncertainty, and concerns regarding treatment efficacy, metastasis, and the impact on one's life. Patients may experience isolation, inadequate support, and additional stressors such as infertility, childcare, marital strain, unemployment, and medical expenses.

Breast care nurses are highly skilled professionals who offer compassionate and comprehensive support to patients at every stage of their journey, from diagnosis and treatment to rehabilitation, symptom management, and survivorship. They serve as the primary point of contact within the multidisciplinary team, ensuring

S.-Y. M. Hung (✉) · A. Yip
S.K. Yee School of Health Sciences, Saint Francis University,
Tseung Kwan O, HKSAR, China
e-mail: syhung@sfu.edu.hk; khyip@sfu.edu.hk

K.-Y. Wong
United Christian Hospital, Kwun Tong, HKSAR, China
e-mail: wongky8@ha.org.hk

that team members are informed about any changes in the patients' health. Key aspects of the breast care nurse's role include providing accurate and up-to-date information, delivering supportive and continuous care, coordinating with the multidisciplinary team, advocating for patients, and promoting self-management and empowerment. Additionally, they assist patients in navigating intimacy issues following mastectomy and managing upper limb lymphedema. Their role is vital in enhancing the quality of life for patients and their families during challenging times. This chapter highlights the professional, comprehensive, and compassionate assistance and support that breast care nurses provide to patients and their families, attending to their needs throughout the course of illness. By examining the multifaceted roles of breast care nurses within an academic setting, this chapter highlights their vital contributions to handling breast disease and improving patient outcomes.

Health Information Needs of Breast Cancer Patients and Survivors

Breast cancer is a disease that affects millions of women worldwide. It is characterized by the abnormal growth of atypical breast cells, which can form tumors. These tumors may be benign (noncancerous) or malignant (cancerous) and can spread to adjacent lymph nodes and metastasize to other organs in the body (World Health Organization 2025b). Treatment strategies for breast cancer vary depending on the type and stage of the disease, often involving a combination of medication, surgery, and radiation therapy. With the rapid development of technology, many individuals seek health information online or through social media. However, alongside factual information, patients may also encounter myths or misconceptions about breast cancer and its management, sometimes propagated by peers or social media. Traditional beliefs, religious views, and misunderstandings regarding the disease can hinder accurate diagnosis and contribute to increased burdens on the healthcare system (Khan et al. 2023). Breast cancer impacts not only the individual's daily life and future lifestyle but also places significant emotional and financial strain on their families and society as a whole.

Breast cancer nurses play a vital role in providing accurate and up-to-date information to patients, helping them navigate the arduous journey of treatment and recovery (Yip et al. 2023). One of their primary responsibilities is to meet the health information needs of breast cancer patients, ensuring that patient-centered care services are delivered effectively (Son et al. 2023). An umbrella review analyzed 14 systematic reviews and identified the major health information needs of breast cancer survivors, which consisted of the three top-ranked information needs related to treatment, supportive care, and body image/sexuality (Gavili et al. 2024). Others included rehabilitation, prognosis, cancer-specific surveillance, health, medical system, coping with cancer, interpersonal, social, financial, and legal information. The research evidence highlights that breast cancer has various physical, psychological, and social impacts on the health of women diagnosed with it, rather than affecting only a specific body organ, the breast.

Supportive Care Needs

Given the intricate features of cancer treatment, it has a significant influence on the daily life of cancer patients and their families, resulting in the need for comprehensive supportive care for well-being (Evans Webb et al. 2021). Supportive care needs may consist of information, emotional, spiritual, social, and physical needs (Evans Webb et al. 2021; Gavili et al. 2024; Yip et al. 2023). Breast care nurses have a fundamental obligation to provide supportive care to breast cancer patients and survivors. Breast cancer patients may experience shock or emotional instability initially due to the uneasy acceptance of the diagnosis (Leão et al. 2022). The patients often have difficulty concentrating on the information provided right after receiving the bad news of their diagnosis, as their denial response influences their cognitive ability temporarily. Nurses should be mindful of the patients' emotional states and address their concerns before conveying any information. Providing information at the appropriate time is imperative (Oakley and Ream 2024). Before initiating communication, it is essential to review the patient's medical records to gain a deeper understanding of their situation, which facilitates empathy and builds rapport (Oakley and Ream 2024). Low mood, fear, and anxiety are common emotions associated with cancer and its treatment. Patients expressed fear of cancer relapse and spread to other organs preoperatively or postoperatively, which was commonly reported in the literature (Leão et al. 2022). Breast care nurses should offer a compassionate presence, provide hope, and deliver essential information clearly and concisely to help alleviate the patients' immediate distress.

Indeed, care provided by breast cancer nurses not only supports the patients but also extends to their families (Franklin et al. 2022; Gavili et al. 2024). Because of the long-lasting duration of breast cancer management with the intricacy of care and challenging psychosocial demands, breast cancer nurses should maintain supportive, respectful, and efficient health care relationships with patients and their families (Franklin et al. 2022; Yip et al. 2023). With the continuity care and support of nurses and families, breast cancer patients receive essential physical, emotional, and psychosocial support during their diagnosis, treatment, and rehabilitation. This assistance helps them regain confidence and reduces feelings of suffering and helplessness, ultimately empowering patients to navigate their cancer treatment journey successfully (Leão et al. 2022).

Coordinating Patient Care with the Multidisciplinary Team

In recent decades, a multidisciplinary team approach has been utilized to provide collaborative and optimal care for cancer patients, including those with breast cancer (Shao et al. 2019). This team typically comprises a diverse range of health-care professionals, including breast surgeons, reconstructive surgeons, radiologists, pathologists, medical oncologists, radiation oncologists, breast care nurses, physiotherapists, psychologists, and social workers. Breast care nurses often serve as the central coordinators within the multidisciplinary team. They facilitate effective communication and collaboration among team members, ensuring seamless integration of care. Additionally, breast care nurses are frequently the primary point of contact for patients and their families. This unique position allows them to gain a deeper understanding of the patient's concerns, priorities, needs, and preferences.

Given the complexity of breast cancer diagnosis and treatment, breast care nurses play a crucial role in conveying the patient's wishes and needs to the multidisciplinary team. They make sure that the patient's voice is heard and that their preferences are considered when creating the treatment plan. Breast care nurses serve as the primary point of contact for patients and their families. They help organize required tests, treatments, and appointments. By serving as a bridge, they help patients navigate the healthcare system, ensuring they have access to vital resources and support services.

Patients' Advocate

Cancer nurses play a pivotal role in patient advocacy, educating others about the supportive care needs of cancer patients (Franklin et al. 2022) and promoting self-advocacy among cancer patients (Alsbrook et al. 2022). Because of the long period of cancer treatment with the rehabilitation process, patients often encounter substantial challenges in physical and emotional status, resulting in a decrease in quality of life. Being the care coordinator and the advocate of breast cancer patients, breast care nurses need to make sure that patients receive appropriate care at the right moment, thus reducing the caregiving burden for women and their families (Franklin et al. 2022).

Self-advocacy is the cancer patients' crucial capability and skill in facing the dreadful disease and emotional burdens of cancer, which include informed decision-making, establishing strength via connection with others, and efficient communication with healthcare professionals (Hagan et al. 2017). A recent qualitative meta-synthesis of self-advocacy experience among cancer patients identified benefits, challenges, and external environmental support as the three essentials (Lin et al. 2025). The self-advocacy experience benefits patients' confidence and self-management capability. Meanwhile, the cancer patients also encountered challenges such as a lack of awareness and obstacles that hindered their self-advocacy experience. Besides, external environmental support, including the health system and social support, contributes to the development of self-advocacy. The authors recommended that cancer nurses and healthcare professionals can promote patients in raising awareness of the benefits and application of self-advocacy, minimize obstacles and optimize participation, and enhance social awareness and support systems, following their recognition of the cancer patients' self-advocacy experience. Cancer nurses can help patients learn to effectively address disease-related issues and initiate discussions to share their views and needs, thereby encouraging patients to participate closely in the decision-making process with healthcare professionals (Lin et al. 2025).

Foster Self-Management and Empowerment

With the advancement of technology, cancer treatments are rapidly evolving. Present treatment typically involves multifaceted and complex therapy, which can exacerbate the difficulties patients encounter with self-care demands (Oakley and Ream 2024). Cancer nurses play a vital role in helping patients manage the physiological and emotional impacts of cancer and its related treatments. It is essential to provide patients with appropriate and effective education that actively involves them in monitoring their symptoms and managing side effects, thereby ensuring their safety (Oakley and Ream 2024). Cancer nurses may consider the self-management capabilities of patients, including their language comprehension, health history, current status, educational level, and emotional stability, to determine their level of involvement (Oakley and Ream 2024).

Through fostering self-management skills, breast care nurses encourage and enable breast cancer patients to become active partners in their own healthcare. One of the fundamental roles of breast care nurses is to promote patient empowerment. Nurses specializing in breast care can enable patients by equipping them with the essential information, abilities, and self-assurance needed to take an active role in overseeing their health and wellness. They offer specialized education and training on self-care strategies, symptom management, and lifestyle modifications related to their body functions, enabling patients to take a proactive role in their recovery. Breast care nurses empower their patients to manage their health journey and engage actively in their own care by delivering thorough education, encouraging collaborative decision-making, providing emotional support, and promoting patient-centered care.

Apart from fostering and empowering patients to manage their own care, family, friends, and other caregivers are encouraged to assist patients in engaging in self-care or to provide various kinds of support at different stages of the disease journey, for instance, emotional support, physical care, or financial assistance, to accompany patients through their devastating and challenging disease journey, especially when they are physically or emotionally unfit. Through enhanced physiological and emotional well-being, patients who are actively involved may experience positive outcomes and benefits (Oakley and Ream 2024).

Navigating Intimacy After Mastectomy

Cancer diagnosis and treatment can substantially influence women's sexual health and intimacy, resulting in a reduced quality of life during and after recovery (Arthur et al. 2022). For instance, many patients and survivors face changes in their bodies that can affect their self-image and sexual well-being after mastectomy (Arthur et al. 2022; Reese et al. 2022; Sledge et al. 2023). Breasts are often viewed as signs of femininity and sexuality, and their absence or alteration may induce adverse emotions, such as feelings of loss, embarrassment, and helplessness. A qualitative study explored breast cancer patients and their partners' views on sexual and intimacy changes (Reese et al. 2022). The study found that breast cancer survivors faced significant concerns, including loss of sexual interest, vaginal discomfort, feelings of guilt about engaging in sexual activities with partners, and the impact of their illness on sexual intimacy within their relationships (Reese et al. 2022). Additionally, patients and their partners expressed a need for more information about the nature and treatment options for the disease.

Similarly, another systematic review analyzed 18 studies of breast cancer survivors' experiences of women of color regarding sexual health and intimacy after cancer treatment (Arthur et al. 2022). The review concluded that the changes in intimacy and sexual health after breast cancer management include mostly negative treatment impacts on sexual health and body image; the gradual process in accepting and overcoming treatment-related changes requires time and perseverance, support socially and spiritually, the significance of positive engagement and encouraging partners, and barriers to sexual health-seeking behaviors and health literacy.

Breast care nurses play a crucial role in helping patients rediscover their sexual interest. This process begins by restoring their self-esteem and allowing them to express their feelings openly and honestly. It involves taking the time to understand their new bodies, reconnecting emotionally and physically, and sharing their feelings with their partners (Reese et al. 2022). Additionally, open communication and interaction can enhance understanding and intimacy, which helps to reduce anxiety regarding sexual issues. Intimacy is not limited to sexual activity. By exploring new forms of intimacy, individuals can navigate this challenging experience and rediscover pleasure in their bodies and relationships.

Navigating Life with Upper Limb Lymphedema After Mastectomy

Breast cancer-related lymphedema, which causes swelling in the upper limb, is a common complication following breast cancer treatment (Zhao et al. 2021). Fatigue and lymphatic pain are also frequent and can be distressing, long-term side effects of breast cancer treatment (Fu et al. 2022). These issues negatively impact the quality of life and physical function of survivors and further hinder their daily activities, contributing to emotional distress and a decline in overall well-being among breast cancer patients. While various conservative treatments exist for breast cancer-related lymphedema—such as compression garments, physiotherapy, and exercise—effective self-management of this condition is essential for overall treatment (Piller 2022). Healthcare professionals and breast care nurses should equip patients with knowledge, educational programs, and holistic support to help them recognize symptoms early and seek timely interventions (Zhao et al. 2021; Piller 2022).

Research has shown that education about lymphedema, its risk factors, skin care, and a home-based exercise program can significantly improve symptoms, including arm tightness, numbness, arm volume, upper extremity function, and overall quality of life in breast cancer patients (Gençay Can et al. 2019). Adjusting to upper limb lymphedema following a mastectomy takes time and involves making changes in daily life. Breast cancer survivors are encouraged to embrace this journey by exploring new activities or interests that work within their physical limitations.

Care for Benign Breast Disease

Most abnormal lesions found in the breast are benign, but they can cause worry and fear among patients (Mau 2018; Thill 2018). Radiologists, oncologists, and pathologists play key roles in distinguishing between benign and malignant breast conditions (Thill 2018). To confirm a diagnosis of benign breast disease, healthcare providers assess the patient's medical history and conduct breast examinations, including physical assessments and radiological imaging. These evaluations help determine the patient's risk of developing breast cancer (Mau 2018; Thill 2018). The risk of breast cancer significantly increases if close relatives have had the disease (Cancer Expert Working Group on Cancer Prevention and Screening (CEWG), Centre for Health Protection, June 2020). Other risk factors include advancing age and a personal history of breast or ovarian cancer. Common signs and symptoms include breast pain, lumps, and abnormal discharge from the nipple; however, some patients may not exhibit any noticeable changes (Mau 2018).

In addition to breast cancer care, breast care nurses play an essential role in managing benign breast conditions and promoting breast health. For instance, breast care nurses support patients dealing with symptoms such as mastalgia (breast pain) and collaborate closely with lactation consultants to assist breastfeeding mothers, especially in cases involving lactational breast abscesses. They also work with other healthcare professionals to educate the community about breast health, promote awareness of breast diseases, and conduct regular screenings and risk assessments. These efforts are crucial for early prevention and identification of breast diseases, ultimately improving the chances for successful treatment and survival (Cancer Expert Working Group on Cancer Prevention and Screening (CEWG), Centre for Health Protection, June 2020).

Conclusion

Breast cancer is the most commonly diagnosed cancer and the leading cause of cancer-related deaths among women worldwide. Millions of women have been affected in the past, and this trend is expected to rise in the coming years. Patients and survivors often face negative consequences. Early detection, combined with advanced surgical treatments and oncological interventions, is crucial for improving survival rates. Breast care nurses are uniquely qualified to provide professional, compassionate, and comprehensive support to patients at every stage of their breast cancer journey. As the initial contact within the multidisciplinary team, they ensure that any changes in patients' health are communicated effectively to all team members. The essential roles of breast cancer nurses include providing accurate health information, delivering supportive and continuous care, coordinating with the multidisciplinary team, advocating for patients, promoting self-management and empowerment, and helping patients navigate challenges such as upper limb lymphedema and intimacy issues following mastectomy. Through collaborative efforts, breast care nurses enhance the quality of life for patients and their families during difficult times.

References

Alsbrook KE, Donovan HS, Wesmiller SW, Thomas TH (2022) Oncology nurses' role in promoting patient self-advocacy. Clin J Oncol Nurs 26(3):239. https://doi.org/10.1188/22.CJON.239-243

Arthur EK, Bissram J, Rechenberg K, Wills A, Campanelli K, Menon U, Nolan TS (2022) Sexual health and intimacy after cancer treatment in women of color: a systematic review. Psycho-Oncology 31(10):1637–1650. https://doi.org/10.1002/pon.6005

Cancer Expert Working Group on Cancer Prevention and Screening (CEWG), Centre for Health Protection (2020) Recommendations on prevention and screening for breast cancer for health professionals, 2020 June

Centre of Health Protection, HKSAR (24 February 2025) https://www.chp.gov.hk/en/healthtopics/content/25/53.html

Devi S (2025) Projected global rise in breast cancer incidence and mortality by 2050. Lancet Oncol 26(4):417. https://doi.org/10.1016/S1470-2045(25)00136-6

Evans Webb M, Murray E, Younger ZW, Goodfellow H, Ross J (2021) The supportive care needs of cancer patients: a systematic review. J Cancer Educ 36(5):899–908. https://doi.org/10.1007/s13187-020-01941-9

Franklin M, Townsend J, Lewis S, Boyle F, Warren M, Ernst K et al (2022) The role and value of metastatic breast care nurses: supporting women and their families to live well with metastatic breast cancer

Fu MR, McTernan ML, Qiu JM, Miaskowski C, Conley YP, Ko E et al (2022) Co-occurring fatigue and lymphatic pain incrementally aggravate their negative effects on activities of daily living, emotional distress, and overall health of breast cancer patients. Integr Cancer Ther 21:15347354221089605. https://doi.org/10.1177/15347354221089605

Gavili N, Sedghi S, Panahi S, Razmgir M (2024) Health information needs of breast cancer survivors: an umbrella review. Breast J 2024(1):5889622. https://doi.org/10.1155/2024/5889622

Gençay Can A, Ekşioğlu E, Çakçı FA (2019) Early detection and treatment of subclinical lymphedema in patients with breast cancer. Lymphat Res Biol 17(3):368–373. https://doi.org/10.1089/lrb.2018.0033

Hagan TL, Rosenzweig MQ, Zorn KK, van Londen GJ, Donovan HS (2017) Perspectives on self-advocacy: comparing perceived uses, benefits, and drawbacks among survivors and providers. Oncol Nurs Forum 44(1):52. https://doi.org/10.1188/17.ONF.52-59

International Agency for Research on Cancer, World Health Organization (2025) Breast cancer. https://www.iarc.who.int/cancer-type/breast-cancer/

Khan S, Jalees S, Jabeen Z, Khan M, Qadri RH, Adnan H et al (2023) Myths and misconceptions of breast cancer in the Pakistani population. Cureus 15(6). https://doi.org/10.7759/cureus.40086

Leão DCM, Pereira ER, Silva RMC, Rocha RCN, Cruz-Quintana F, García-Caro MP (2022) Spiritual and emotional experience with a diagnosis of breast cancer: a scoping review. Cancer Nurs 45(3):224–235. https://doi.org/10.1097/NCC.0000000000000936

Lin L, Jin Y, Feng C, Zhu K (2025) The experience of self-advocacy among cancer patients: a qualitative meta-synthesis. PLoS One 20(4):e0321719. https://doi.org/10.1371/journal.pone.0321719

Mau K (2018) Benign breast diseases: an introduction for the advanced practice nurse. Clin J Oncol Nurs 22(5):493–495. https://doi.org/10.1188/18.cjon.493-495

Oakley, C., & Ream, E. (2024). Role of the nurse in patient education and engagement and its importance in advanced breast cancer. In Seminars in oncology nursing (40, 1, 151556). WB Saunders. doi:https://doi.org/10.1016/j.soncn.2023.151556

Piller NB (2022) Recognition of those at risk of lymphedema, benefits of subclinical detection, and the importance of targeted treatment and management. Indian J Vasc Endovasc Surg 9(3):215–222. https://doi.org/10.4103/ijves.ijves_33_22

Reese JB, Zimmaro LA, McIlhenny S, Sorice K, Porter LS, Zaleta AK et al (2022) Coping with changes to sex and intimacy after a diagnosis of metastatic breast cancer: results from a qualitative investigation with patients and partners. Front Psychol 13:864893. https://doi.org/10.3389/fpsyg.2022.864893

Shao J, Rodrigues M, Corter AL, Baxter NN (2019) Multidisciplinary care of breast cancer patients: a scoping review of multidisciplinary styles, processes, and outcomes. Curr Oncol 26(3):e385. https://doi.org/10.3747/co.26.4713

Sledge P, Friedman A, Champagne AM (2023) Beauty, breasts, and meaning after mastectomy. In: Interpreting the body, 1st edn. Bristol University Press, pp 133–154. https://doi.org/10.51952/9781529211580.ch006

Son NT, Hsin-Tien HSU, Huong PTT, Trung TQ (2023) Information needs of patients with breast cancer undergoing treatment in Vietnam and related determinants. J Nurs Res 31(2):e265. https://doi.org/10.1097/jnr.0000000000000546

Thill M (2018) Benign breast diseases. Breast Care 13(6):400–401

World Health Organization (2025a) Cancer. https://www.who.int/news-room/fact-sheets/detail/cancer

World Health Organization (2025b) Breast cancer. https://www.who.int/news-room/fact-sheets/detail/breast-cancer

Yip KH, Yip YC, Tsui WK, Chan CS, Mo YH, Smith GD (2023) Navigating changes: a qualitative study exploring the health-related quality of breast cancer survivors during the coronavirus disease 2019 pandemic. J Adv Nurs 80(4):1243–1665. https://doi.org/10.1111/jan.15909

Zhao H, Wu Y, Zhou C, Li W, Li X, Chen L (2021) Breast cancer-related lymphedema patient and healthcare professional experiences in lymphedema self-management: a qualitative study. Support Care Cancer 29:8027–8044. https://doi.org/10.1007/s00520-021-06390-8

An Exploration of Brain Death, Organ Donation, and the Essential Role of Organ Donation Coordinators in Hong Kong

Suk-Man Cheung, Alice Yip, and Yu-Tim Leung

Introduction: The Origin and Evolution of Organ Transplant in Hong Kong

The history of organ transplantation in Hong Kong comprises significant milestones over the years. In 1961, Tung Wah Eastern Hospital witnessed the first corneal transplant in Hong Kong, marking a pioneering step. The late 1960s saw the inaugural homologous kidney transplantation at Queen Mary Hospital (QMH) in 1969. Notably, 1991 witnessed a series of breakthroughs at QMH, including the first homologous liver transplantation and bone transplant. The subsequent year, 1992, featured the first homologous heart transplantation at Grantham Hospital (GH), along with the first skin transplant. In 1995, GH achieved another milestone with the first homologous single lung transplant and combined heart-lung transplant. The progress continued in 1997 with the first double-lung transplant at GH. Subsequently, years witnessed advancements in complex transplant procedures. Notably, QMH performed the first combined liver-kidney transplant in 2001, followed by the first combined heart-liver transplant in 2010.

S.-M. Cheung (✉) · Y.-T. Leung
Hospital Authority, Kowloon, HKSAR, China
e-mail: csm714@ha.org.hk; lyt187@ha.org.hk

A. Yip
School of Health Sciences, St. Francis University,
Tseung Kwan O, Hong Kong
e-mail: khyip@sfu.edu.hk

The Development of Organ Donation Coordination Service

The development of the organ donation coordination service in Hong Kong is marked by crucial phases. Before the establishment of the Transplant Coordination Service, medical professionals, including intensivists and critical care physicians, undertook coordination responsibilities within their hospitals. In August 1988, the first Transplant Coordination Centre emerged at QMH, initially overseen by the Hospital Service Department. By 1994, a total of four full-time equivalent organ transplant coordinators were stationed across renal transplant hospitals. The late 2000s saw the establishment of Cluster Coordinating Committees for Transplant Service within each of the seven clusters. These committees were formed to enhance coordination, ensure regulatory compliance, and raise awareness of organ donation. Notably, in 2016, the role name transitioned from "transplant coordinator" to "organ donation coordinator (ODC)" to align with the evolving focus on organ donation efforts. Presently, nine full-time ODCs cater to the entire population of 7.5 million Hong Kong citizens, extending their services to all hospitals, both public and private (Legislative Council of the Government of the Hong Kong Special Administrative Region (HKSAR) 2016).

Opt-in System in Hong Kong

Hong Kong's organ donation policy follows an "opt-in" system, where individuals are required to explicitly express their wish for organ donation before it can be carried out posthumously (Zeng et al. 2023). Despite efforts to increase awareness, the organ donation rate in Hong Kong, while comparatively high in Asia at 4.66 donors per million population in 2022, remains lower than rates in Western countries like the United States, the United Kingdom, and Spain (Legislative Council HKSAR 2023).

Several factors contribute to the challenges faced by organ donation efforts in Hong Kong. Chinese cultural beliefs, including the importance of keeping the body intact after death, pose a significant obstacle. Moreover, some individuals may have expressed objections to organ donation while alive, adding to the complexity. The uncertainty about the wishes of the deceased further complicates the decision-making process for families.

The Development of Centralized Organ Donation Register (CODR)

In 2008, Hong Kong introduced the CODR to streamline the organ donation registration process (Department of Health 2008). By 31 May 2025, more than 400,982 Hong Kong residents had registered their thoughts with CODR (Department of Health 2025). However, despite these initiatives, the consent rate for organ donation has remained relatively static at 40–50%, reflecting the persistent challenges.

Comparatively, other countries have adopted different organ donation policies. Some countries, like Spain, follow an "opt-out" system, where individuals are presumed to consent to organ donation unless they explicitly state otherwise (Legislative Council HKSAR 2016). This approach has contributed to higher donation rates in certain regions. Understanding the cultural, societal, and legal dynamics surrounding organ donation policies is crucial for addressing challenges and devising strategies to enhance organ donation rates in Hong Kong. Balancing cultural sensitivities with effective communication and education initiatives may play a key role in fostering a supportive environment for organ donation (Li et al. 2019).

Stressors Faced by Families of Imminent Brain-Dead Organ Donors

False Hope of Family's Misinterpretation from Readings

The hospital equipment produces both normal operational sounds and alarms, which may be unfamiliar and unsettling to family members of an impending brain-dead patient. Some individuals may experience fear or interpret the alarms as indicative of danger or malevolence. Additionally, there is a tendency for misinterpretation of monitor readings, as family members may place hope in the displayed lines, waves, or numerical values without a comprehensive understanding. This misinterpretation may lead to false optimism, overlooking the irreversible trauma or stroke that has rendered the patient in an unsalvageable state. Afterall, they tend to neglect all the negative things or feelings, instead they try to look up for positive ones. They are unwilling to receive any bad news from health care professionals. The conversation with a family member:

> Family member: "Doctor, is my older brother's condition improving?"
> Doctor: "No, his condition remains critical."
> Family member: "That's not right! The blood pressure displayed on the monitor appears normal."
> Doctor: "We've increased his dosage of cardiotonic medications to maintain his current blood pressure."
> Family member: "That's incorrect. His current blood pressure readings are significantly improved compared to those from this morning. Do you concur?"
> Doctor: "That's a plausible interpretation."
> Family member: "Consequently, there has been a positive change in my brother's condition."

Facing the realities of a loved one's illness presents a formidable challenge for families. Frequently, as a coping mechanism, they may selectively attend to positive information provided by healthcare professionals, thereby maintaining a sense of hope.

However, it is crucial for families to directly address the realities of the situation. While potentially distressing, comprehending the accurate trajectory of the illness facilitates informed decision-making and ensures the patient receives appropriate care and support.

Encouraging families to acknowledge the reality of their loved one's condition, even when distressing, facilitates more effective navigation of the complexities of healthcare and ultimately establishes a foundation for more effective coping and support strategies. By fostering open and honest communication, healthcare professionals can empower families to face impending challenges with great resilience.

Role Confusion Between Organ Donation Coordinator (ODC) and Medical Officer

Families sometimes mistakenly perceive ODCs as medical officers (doctors), particularly when ODCs explain the patient's critical condition. The pronouncement of ODCs appears to carry significant weight. Consequently, when requesting consent for organ donation, families tend to readily accept and comprehend the information presented by ODCs, ultimately facilitating informed decision-making regarding the patient's care. A conversation between the patient's son and the ODC:

Patient's son:	"I understand my father's condition is critical. I am prepared for the possibility of his imminent passing."
ODC:	"You are correct. His respiration, heartbeat, and blood pressure are currently being maintained artificially through mechanical ventilation and pharmacological intervention. Physicians have administered medication to manage diabetes insipidus, and nursing staff are utilizing warming blankets to regulate his body temperature. Clinically, he meets the criteria for brain death; however, confirmatory testing by a physician is required."
Patient's son:	"Doctor, the situation is far more serious than I realized."
ODC:	"I am not a medical doctor (medical officer)."
Patient's son:	"Understood. Should my father pass away, would organ donation be a possibility? I am concerned that his advanced age might pose a contraindication."
ODC:	"Age is not necessarily a limiting factor. Ultimately, the suitability for organ donation will be by physician assessment and diagnostic testing."
Patient's son:	"Kindly request a doctor's assessment of my father's suitable as an organ donor."

When families misunderstand the roles of healthcare professionals, it is essential to provide clarification while maintaining a respectful and empathetic approach. Promoting a comprehensive understanding of the diverse roles within the healthcare system and the collaborative nature of patient care is crucial. This includes highlighting the distinct contributions of each professional and emphasizing the importance of interprofessional collaboration for optimal patient outcomes. It is important to facilitate familial understanding of the distinct yet complementary roles within the healthcare team. While physicians typically focus on diagnosis and treatment planning, nurses provide essential hands-on patient care, including monitoring patient progress and offering emotional support. Furthermore, adequate time should be allowed for families to acclimate to the roles of various healthcare professionals, particularly in life-or-death situations. Consistent and clear communication regarding the responsibilities of each team member is vital.

Challenges in Identifying Consistent Caregivers

The three-shift duty roster, which governs the rotating schedules of healthcare personnel such as nurses and physicians, often results in varying staff presence and attire. Consequently, family members may experience challenges identifying the designated caregivers for their relatives, leading to confusion when seeking assistance. This can contribute to perceptions of inadequate support and a lack of empathy from healthcare professionals. Conversely, providers perceive family requests as excessive or redundant.

The Impact of Visitation Restrictions on Donor Families' Grieving Process

Restrictions on visiting hours for families of potential organ donors, particularly during the coronavirus disease (COVID-19) pandemic (Low 2020), profoundly affected their ability to process grief and express emotions following the declaration of brain death. These limitations deprived families of valuable opportunities for closure and final farewells during an acutely distressing period. The inability to be physically present with their loved ones exacerbated emotional suffering, compounding the already complex grieving process (Tsui et al. 2023). Furthermore, providing designated spaces and resources for donor families to express their emotions is essential. The following dialogue took place between a nurse and the husband of a potential organ donor during the COVID-19 pandemic:

> Husband: (Standing at the ward entrance with an iPad) "My love, do not worry about us. Be at peace. The children and I are here, just outside. We are unable to come in right now due to the restrictions, allowing only one visit per person per day. We'll come in to say our final goodbyes when they pronounce you … Nurse, would it be possible to make an exception and allow us to come in? My wife is expected to be declared brain dead today."
>
> Nurse: "I am very sorry, but that's not possible. Due to the severity of the COVID-19 situation, we must strictly adhere to ward regulations."

Utilizing video conferencing technology, such as iPads or similar devices, facilitates virtual presence at the bedside, offering a valuable alternative to physical presence during times of restricted access. While not a substitute for in-person connection, this technology enables families to maintain visual and auditory contact with their loved ones, providing crucial opportunities for emotional expression, sharing memories, and final farewells. This real-time interaction can offer solace and foster a sense of connection, potentially mitigating the emotional burden during an exceptionally challenging period.

The Burden of Decision-Making in Brainstem Death Testing

In clinical practice, the decision to conduct brainstem death testing rests with medical professionals. However, during family interviews, physicians, driven by empathy, may inadvertently engage in discussions regarding the timing and appropriateness of such testing. While intended to demonstrate empathy and respect for family autonomy, this approach can inadvertently shift the burden of decision-making onto family members, requiring them to determine the timing to confirm their loved one's death. Consequently, some families may decline brainstem death testing, perceiving it as a decisive act in ending their loved one's life, rather than a confirmatory medical procedure. This reluctance stems not from a misunderstanding of the concept of brain death but from the emotional difficulty of authorizing a procedure that formally acknowledges the irreversible loss of their loved one. The following dialogue transpired between a physician and the son of a potential organ donor:

> Physician: "Today, we need to perform two sets of tests to confirm brain death in your mother."
>
> Son: "Today? Is it possible to postpone this?"
>
> Physician: "Please take some time to discuss with your family when you would prefer us to conduct the tests. After the two rounds of testing are complete, we will ensure your mother is comfortable and withdraw any medications and life support that are no longer needed."
>
> Son: "I cannot consent to the tests. I am not prepared for my mother to die." (The son was observed to be crying uncontrollably.)

The decision to perform brainstem death testing is a clinical judgment made by physicians based on the patient's condition and established medical criteria. This critical determination is guided by the patient's best interests and adheres to established medical protocols and ethical guidelines (Food and Health Bureau 2017). It is important to emphasize that this clinical decision is not subject to family consent. Therefore, clear, compassionate, and comprehensive communication with the patient's family is essential prior to brainstem death testing. Families should receive detailed information regarding the patient's clinical status, the diagnostic criteria for brain death, and the procedures involved in the testing process.

The Complexities of Organ Donation Consent

The decision to consent to organ donation presents complex emotional and practical considerations for families facing bereavement. This decision can be particularly stressful, often involving a conflict between the altruistic desire to help others in need and uncertainty regarding the deceased's wishes. Furthermore, families may encounter resistance from elderly relatives or other close family members due to religious or traditional beliefs. Concerns about potential postmortem disfigurement can further exacerbate the family's distress. The conversation between the ODC and the potential donor's son is documented below:

> ODC: "Would you consider authorizing organ donation for your mother?"
>
> Son: "She never discussed it. I am unsure of her wishes. She was always very concerned about her appearance, so I am worried about potential disfigurement. I also do not know how my grandparents and other relatives will react. My mother was religious; I am not sure if this will affect her afterlife."
>
> ODC: "You could make the decision based on your understanding of your mother's character and values."
>
> Son: "This is a very difficult decision."

In navigating these multifaceted concerns, healthcare professionals play a pivotal role in providing families with comprehensive information, support, and guidance. This includes addressing any misconceptions, respecting cultural and religious sensitivities, and offering reassurance regarding the preservation of the deceased's physical appearance following organ donation. Ultimately, facilitating open and empathetic communication empowers families to make informed decisions that align with their values and the deceased's wishes while also recognizing the profound impact organ donation can have on the lives of others.

Incentives and Disincentives for Organ Donation: A Comparison

The absence of financial incentives, such as support for funeral expenses, in Hong Kong may present a challenge to promoting organ donation (Chow et al. 2022). Some jurisdictions offer incentives to encourage organ donation. In South Korea, for example, the government provides a funeral allowance to the next of kin of deceased donors. Taiwan prioritizes individuals on organ waiting lists if a family member has previously donated an organ. Conversely, Hong Kong primarily offers nonfinancial incentives, such as a commemorative plaque in a remembrance park managed by the Board of Management of the Chinese Permanent Cemeteries and a certificate of appreciation from the Hospital Authority. An experienced ODC conversed with the potential donor's brother-in-law, a visitor from South Korea:

Brother-in-law:	"Is there any financial assistance available for funeral expenses if my brother-in-law becomes an organ donor?"
ODC:	"In Hong Kong, organ donation is considered an altruistic act. Therefore, no financial incentives, such as monetary compensation for the deceased's family, are provided."

Post-death Adjustment and Coping

Families face challenges adjusting to life after the death of a relative, including forming post-death bonds with the deceased and adapting to a world without their loved one. Bereaved families who altruistically donate the organs of their deceased loved ones may find peace in contemplating an afterlife, often envisioning a serene heavenly existence. However, contrasted with this comforting image, they may also reflect upon the organ procurement process itself, potentially harboring anxieties regarding its perceived impact on their loved one's postmortem spiritual journey. These complex emotions often arise from deeply rooted cultural and religious beliefs and intuitive spiritual sensibilities.

Case One Mothers who have donated their children's organs.

> Mother: "What is the surgical process for organ donation?"
> ODC: "To organ procurement, the organs are cooled in situ by packing the abdominal cavity with crushed ice."
> Mother: "In my dream, my child told me her stomach was cold."

Case Two

A poignant narrative details a dinner with a bereaved family, in which the wife recounted her decision to authorize the donation of her husband's organs. The deceased's second wife found the dinner provided a safe environment to articulate her anxieties regarding future relationships with her stepdaughters. This interaction offered significant emotional support and emotional release, facilitating authentic self-expression.

Following a successful organ donation case, donor families often experience a protracted bereavement period. ODCs provide ongoing psychosocial support, empathetically engaging with the families' joys and concerns, thereby fostering a strong rapport. However, constrained by their primary clinical nursing responsibilities, coordinators cannot fully function as social workers or clinical psychologists. This intrinsic limitation can pose significant challenges and stressors for donor families. Nevertheless, ODCs endeavor to offer compassionate companionship and support, similar to a shared journey of life alongside the family (Dicks et al. 2023).

Informed Decision-Making Hurdles

Families facing the challenge of limited brain death awareness often experience significant difficulty navigating organ donation decisions. This lack of understanding can contribute to reluctance or refusal to consent to donation, stemming from an incomplete comprehension of brain death's irreversibility. A dialogue between an ODC and a husband experiencing psychological resistance to organ donation is presented below:

Husband:	"I consent to the donation of my wife's organs. Following the cessation of her heartbeat, will she be transferred to the mortuary for organ procurement?"
ODC:	"That is incorrect. Mechanical and pharmacological support will maintain your wife's heartbeats until the organ procurement procedure is completed in the operating room." (The husband paused in thoughtful consideration)
Husband:	"I understand that my wife is brainstem dead, but I am unable to accept organ procurement prior to cessation of cardiac activity."
ODC:	"Upon cessation of cardiac function and the subsequent circulatory arrest, organs rapidly deteriorate, rendering them unsuitable for transplantation. Consequently, only corneal and skin donation would be feasible."

Public education regarding brain death is essential to address widespread misconceptions and the frequent conflation of brain death with legal death. This lack of understanding can hinder informed decision-making regarding organ donation during critical periods. To address this issue, media platforms such as television, YouTube, Facebook, and Instagram can be utilized to disseminate accurate information regarding brain death. Furthermore, engaging experts in public discussions about brain death can enhance understanding of this complex concept.

Additionally, the Hong Kong government could strengthen these efforts by implementing online and media campaigns, community outreach programs, and educational workshops and seminars. These initiatives would reinforce public understanding of brain death and facilitate consideration of organ donation. Increased awareness of the equivalence of brain death and legal death may increase the likelihood of families consenting to donation.

Cultural and Religious Beliefs in Conflict with Organ Donation Practices

Families may experience conflicts between personal beliefs and values, particularly when cultural or religious perspectives on death and organ donation are ambiguous or poorly understood. Such conflicts can create disagreement among family members, hindering consensus regarding organ donation decisions.

Case Three

A leading figure within a Buddhist lineage:	"According to our doctrines, the cranial surgery performed on your husband is not permissible."
The potential donor's wife:	"The urgency of the situation prompted me to make this ill-advised decision."
ODC:	"Would you consider authorizing organ donation for your husband? Many religious faiths regard saving lives as an act of immense merit."
The potential donor's wife	"While I generally support organ donation, I cannot consider it if the procedure would in any way comprise my husband's passage into the afterlife."

Case Four

ODC:	"Will you be making the decision regarding organ donation for the patient?"
Family member 1:	"We are unaware of the patient's wishes regarding organ donation, therefore, making a decision on his behalf is challenging."
Family member 2:	"We are apprehensive about making an incorrect decision, fearing potential negative repercussions, both real and perceived, should the patient's wishes have been misinterpreted."

During the interview, ODCs provide factual information regarding the organ donation process, including its compatibility with various religious perspectives. Coordinators demonstrate respect for cultural and religious beliefs by acknowledging their significance in the decision-making process. Illustrative examples of religious support for organ donation are offered. Finally, ODCs recognize the profound personal nature of organ donation decisions and uphold the autonomy of each family member. They emphasize that the decision is not about right or wrong but rather about aligning with the values and beliefs of the potential donor and their family.

No Consensus among the Family

When families experience conflict and cannot reach a consensus regarding organ donation, the process cannot proceed. This inability to reach agreement constitutes a significant stressor for family members, often necessitating extensive deliberation. The following presents the family discussion regarding organ donation for their deceased loved one:

> Father: "I dissent from the donation of my son's organs. I have received no communication regarding his decision to donate his organs. Further elaboration is unnecessary."
>
> Sister: "My elder brother once expressed to me his thoughts on organ donation."
>
> Mother: "I wish to fulfil my son's final wishes."
>
> Maternal uncle: "While my brother-in-law and I share a disapproval of organ donation, I nevertheless wish to honor my nephew's final request in this matter."
>
> [After a period of protracted consideration, father ultimately consented to sign the organ donation authorization form]

ODCs play a crucial role in facilitating discussions among family members regarding organ donation. They can provide information, address concerns, and guide the conversation in a positive and respectful manner. If the deceased has not previously discussed organ donation with their family, ODCs should encourage the family to consider the deceased's personality, values, and beliefs when deciding.

If the deceased had expressed a wish to donate organs, this should be respected and emphasized during discussions with the family. Highlighting the importance of honoring their autonomous decision serves to respect their memory and legacy. Should disagreements persist, facilitating productive discussions can help the family reach a consensus. Offering a neutral perspective can guide the family toward a decision that respects everyone's viewpoints. Ultimately, the autonomy of each family member in the decision-making process must be respected.

Time Makes Organ Donation Possible

Timely decision-making regarding organ donation can be challenging for bereaved families, particularly when certain factors are present. The absence of explicit directives from the deceased regarding organ donation introduces complexity to the process. Consultation with multiple family members can further prolong the decision timeline. Moreover, the emotional burden of grief, often exacerbated by exhaustion and distress, can hinder prompt decision-making.

After a 13-year-old girl was declared brain dead, ODC inquired whether the girl's mother would consider donating her daughter's organ.

Mother: "I am not prepared to make a decision regarding organ donation at this time. Could I have two more days to spend with my daughter?"

Doctor: "I understand. However, only nutritional support via feeding tube will be provided, while mechanical and pharmacological life support will remain unchanged until Saturday, at which point all life-sustaining interventions will be withdrawn."

Two days later, the family gathered at the patient's bedside to say their final goodbyes.

Sister: "Mother, I dreamt of my sister last night. She told me she wanted to donate her organs to help other."

Mother: "Truly? Please inform the nurse immediately. I wish to proceed with organ donation for my daughter."

Subsequently, the hospital notified ODCs that the patient's mother had reconsidered and wished to proceed with organ donation.

Navigating the time-sensitive nature of organ donation decisions, particularly in cases involving hemodynamically unstable potential donors, necessitates a delicate balance between medical urgency and the family's emotional processing. While time is of the essence, respecting the family's need to process information and arrive at a decision is paramount. Encouraging questions and the open expression of thoughts should be coupled with a sensitive conveyance of the urgency inherent in organ donation.

Conclusion

Organ donation in Hong Kong faces complexities stemming from cultural sensitivities surrounding brain death and the emotional burden on grieving families. ODCs play a vital role in supporting families through the decision-making process, balancing medical urgency with cultural understanding and emotional support to honor autonomous choices.

Acknowledgments   The authors express their gratitude to the family members of deceased organ donors and the healthcare professionals serving on organ donation teams for their contributions to this chapter.

References

Chow, K. M., Ahn, C., Dittmer, I., Au, D. K. S., Cheung, I., Cheng, Y. L., Lau, C. S., Yeung, D., & Li, P. K. T. (2022). Introducing incentives and reducing disincentives in enhancing deceased organ donation and transplantation. In Seminars in nephrology (42, 4, 151268). WB Saunders. https://doi.org/10.1016/j.semnephrol.2022.07.002

Department of Health (2008) Press release: central register set up to facilitate organ donation. The Government of the Hong Kong Special Administrative Region. https://www.dh.gov.hk/english/press/2008/081124.html. Accessed on 30 June 2025

Department of Health (2025) Organ donation: number of registrations recorded in the centralised organ donation register. The Government of the Hong Kong Special Administrative Region. https://www.organdonation.gov.hk/en/. Accessed on 30 June 2025

Dicks SG, Northam HL, van Haren FM, Boer DP (2023) The bereavement experiences of families of potential organ donors: a qualitative longitudinal case study illuminating opportunities for family care. Int J Qual Stud Health Well Being 18(1):2149100. https://doi.org/10.1080/17482631.2022.2149100

Food and Health Bureau (2017) Background information on organ donation and transplant. The Government of the Hong Kong Special Administrative Region. https://www.healthbureau.gov.hk/download/press_and_publications/otherinfo/170600_organ_donation_transplant/e_background_paper_organ_donation_transplant.pdf. Accessed on 30 June 2025

Legislative Council Commission, The Government of the Hong Kong Special Administrative Region (HKSAR) (2016) Organ donation in Hong Kong. The Government of the Hong Kong Special Administrative Region. https://www.legco.gov.hk/research-publications/english/1516rb05-organ-donation-in-hong-kong-20160714-e.pdf. Accessed on 30 June 2025

Legislative Council, HKSAR (2023) LC Paper No. CB(3)670/2023(01). Implementing cooperation with the mainland in organ transplant. The Government of the Hong Kong Special Administrative Region. https://www.legco.gov.hk/yr2023/english/counmtg/motion/cm20230524m-lty-prpt-e.pdf. Accessed on 30 June 2025

Li MT, Hillyer GC, Husain SA, Mohan S (2019) Cultural barriers to organ donation among Chinese and Korean individuals in the United States: a systematic review. Transpl Int 32(10):1001–1018. https://doi.org/10.1111/tri.13439

Low Z (2020) Coronavirus: some Hong Kong hospitals to resume visiting hours for family members next week, as city records no new COVID-19 cases. South China Morning Post. https://sc.mp/dfrx3?utm_source=copy-link&utm_campaign=3088376&utm_medium=share_widget. Accessed on 30 June 2025

Tsui WK, Yip KH, Yip YC (2023) Heartbreak and loneliness due to family separations and limited visiting during COVID-19: a qualitative study. Int J Environ Res Public Health 20(2):1633. https://doi.org/10.3390/ijerph20021633

Zeng M, Li H, Song X, Jiang J, Chen Y (2023) Factors associated with willingness toward organ donation in China: a nationwide cross-sectional analysis using a social–ecological framework. Healthcare 11(6):824. https://doi.org/10.3390/healthcare11060824

Part IV

Care Networks and Trajectories

Advancements in Burn Care and Rehabilitation: A Comprehensive Approach with Global Implications

12

Tze-Wing Wong and Alice Yip

Community Health Education on Burn Prevention and Correct First Aid Treatment

Preventing burn injuries is demonstrably superior to treating them. Community-based educational initiatives focused on burn prevention are therefore critical. In Hong Kong, the majority of burn injuries occur within the home environment. Young children, particularly toddlers, are frequently victims of accidental scalding by hot liquids due to parental or caregiver oversight. Zou et al. (2015) indicate that the majority of pediatric burn injuries occur in or near the home environment, irrespective of the country's development status. Kitchens, living rooms, and bathrooms are frequently cited as the locations of these incidents (Jonsson et al. 2017). However, such accidents are largely preventable. Furthermore, elderly individuals living alone, particularly those with pre-existing medical conditions (comorbidities), constitute a high-risk group for burn and scald injuries. Prompt and appropriate first aid application following a burn or scald injury significantly improves clinical outcomes and wound healing (McLure et al. 2021).

Harish et al. (2019) highlights the established importance of cooling burn wounds with running water to mitigate progressive tissue damage following a burn injury. This practice is crucial for preserving the wound's capacity for reepithelialization and minimizing scar formation. First aid protocols recommend irrigating the burn with cool running water for a minimum of 20 min, ideally within 3 h of the injury

T.-W. Wong (✉)
Prince of Wales Hospital, Shatin, HKSAR, China
e-mail: wtw342@ha.org.hk

A. Yip
School of Health Sciences, St. Francis University,
Tseung Kwan O, Hong Kong
e-mail: khyip@sfu.edu.hk

A. Yip, G. D. Smith (eds.), *Surgical Nursing in Practice*,
https://doi.org/10.1007/978-3-032-14729-5_12

(Burgess et al. 2019; Harish et al. 2019). Subsequent medical evaluation is essential to accurately assess the severity of the burn.

Health education booths focusing on burn prevention and appropriate first aid treatment are featured at the World Health Organization health carnivals and District Health Centers. Public forums addressing home safety and preventative measures against burn and scald incidents are also offered to the community. Furthermore, public service announcements concerning burn prevention and home safety are broadcast on Radio Television Hong Kong to disseminate this crucial information.

Management of Life-Threatening Conditions in Burn Trauma

The management of life-threatening conditions in burn trauma begins with a rapid initial assessment. These protocols are crucial for immediate identification and stabilization of critical issues (Wong et al. 2023). Within Accident and Emergency Departments, these assessment drive triage and evaluation of burn injuries, directing patients to the appropriate care setting, ranging from specialized burn units to outpatient clinics, based on individual needs.

Airway Assessment and Cervical Spine Precautions

Confirmation of a patent airway is essential for assessing patient responsiveness. Cervical spine immobilization with a cervical collar is indicated if cervical spine injury is suspected.

Respiratory Assessment and Oxygen Supplementation

Inhalation of heated gases and smoke during flame burns can cause respiratory tract injury. Direct thermal injury to the upper airways may induce edema formation, potentially leading to airway obstruction. Supplemental oxygen should be administered at a non-rebreather mask at a flow rate of 15 L/min. Pulse oximetry should be monitored continuously. Progressive hoarseness should be considered a significant indicator of impending airway compromise. Respiratory rate, depth, symmetry, and adequate chest expansion should be assessed.

Circulation with Hemorrhage Assessment

Patients should be assessed for hemorrhage and appropriate management initiated. Blood pressure may not be a reliable indicator of hemodynamic status in patients with extensive burns due to the pathophysiological changes and extremity oedema associated with burn injuries. Heart rate is a more useful parameter for evaluating the adequacy of fluid resuscitation. Neurological status should be assessed by evaluating the patient's level of consciousness. Maintain normothermia. Burn extent should be determined using the Lund and Browder chart (Giretzlehner et al. 2021; Kotecha et al. 2022).

A secondary survey should be conducted after initial stabilization and management of life-threatening conditions. This comprehensive assessment should include obtaining a detailed patient history, including past medical history, current medications, allergies, and the circumstances surrounding the injury. Intravenous access should be established, and fluid resuscitation initiated according to established protocols. Tetanus prophylaxis should be updated as indicated. Burn wounds should be covered with appropriate dressings to prevent contamination and provide analgesia. A thorough head-to-toe examination should be performed.

Criteria for Major Burn Injury in Adults and Children

The criteria for defining major burns in adults and children differ due to variations in physiological response and body surface area distribution. Adults with burns covering $\geq 20\%$ of their total body surface area (TBSA) are considered to have major burns. In contrast, children with burns involving $\geq 10\%$ of their TBSA are classified as having major burns (Rossella et al. 2022). This distinction is crucial because children have a higher surface area-to-body mass ratio, making them more susceptible to fluid and heat loss. Consequently, they require more aggressive fluid resuscitation and are at greater risk of complications, such as hypothermia and hypovolemic shock. Furthermore, the immature immune system in children increases their susceptibility to infections following burn injuries. Therefore, specialized pediatric burn care is essential for optimal management.

Laser Doppler Imaging for Burn Depth Assessment

Early diagnosis and accurate assessment of burn wound depth are crucial for optimal burn management. Laser Doppler imaging (LDI) offers a noninvasive, noncontact method for objective and early determination of burn depth and prediction of healing potential. LDI can be effectively utilized between 48 h and 5 days postburn injury, facilitating timely therapeutic intervention and evaluation (Burke-Smith et al. 2015; Wang et al. 2020). This early assessment allows for more informed decisions regarding wound care, surgical requirements (e.g., the need for skin grafting), and overall treatment strategy, potentially minimizing scarring and improving patient outcomes.

Comprehensive training in LDI theory and practice is essential for nurses involved in burn care. This training should encompass proper scanning techniques, accurate interpretation of LDI results, adherence to safety protocols, and recognition and mitigation of confounding factors. The LDI device employs low-power laser light to penetrate the burn wound and detect the movement of red blood cells within the capillaries, arterioles, and venules. This generates a color-coded map representing microcirculatory blood perfusion, enabling differentiation between superficial dermal burns, mid-to-deep dermal burns, and full-thickness burns. This objective assessment facilitates early and targeted burn treatment strategies. The use of LDI for burn depth assessment is supported by evidence and is considered standard practice (Gill 2013; Wang et al. 2020).

Burn Wound Management Strategies

Effective burn wound management is critical for preventing infection and promoting optimal healing. Maintaining hygiene, including hair washing and showering, is essential prior to any wound dressing procedure (Knighton 2020).

Adequate analgesia must be administered prior to burn wound dressing changes. Treatment modalities are determined by the depth of the burn wound. Therapeutic dressings are employed to facilitate epithelialization and optimal wound healing. A superficial dermal burn affects the epidermis and the superficial layer of the dermis. The wound presents with a pinkish appearance, blister formation, brisk capillary refill, and intense pain. A mid-dermal burn exhibits a darker pink coloration compared to a superficial dermal burn. Capillary refill may be sluggish, and while large blisters may still be present and prone to rupture, sensation to touch is diminished, though pain persists.

Superficial and Mid-dermal Burn Wounds

The aims are to promote wound epithelialization and prevent infection. Biological dressings, including porcine skin or human amniotic membrane, are applied to burn wounds to alleviate pain and enhance epithelialization. However, daily monitoring of wound progression is essential. Maceration of biological dressing may occur due to the presence of exudate, necessitating reapplication after wound cleansing. Complete epithelialization of the burn wound is the desired outcome.

A deep dermal burn wound involves the destruction of structures essential for spontaneous healing. The wound presents with a dark red, blotchy appearance, diminished or absent capillary refill, and loss of sensation. The aims are to minimize necrotic tissue formation and prevent wound infection. Initially, the wound is irrigated with a disinfectant solution, such as Granudacyn®, to cleanse the area and inhibit the proliferation of both gram-positive and gram-negative bacteria (Esin et al. 2022). Subsequently, thorough cleansing (debridement performs by physicians) of slough and necrotic tissue is performed by burn nurses, often utilizing UCS™ debridement cloths (Gillies 2019; Mayer et al. 2024). Finally, enzymatic debridement, using agents such as Iruxol® mono ointment, is employed to further remove slough and promote wound healing (Salehi et al. 2020). This multifaceted approach yields significant therapeutic benefits.

In full-thickness burns, both the epidermal and dermal layers of the skin are damaged. The wound appears white, dry, charred, and leathery, with absent capillary refill and sensation. Deeper structures, including subcutaneous fat, tendons, muscle, and bone, may also be involved. Surgical debridement and autologous meshed skin grafting are typically required. The application of skin grafts to full-thickness burns minimizes or prevents hypertrophic scar formation. Burn nurses have developed specialized knowledge and skills in managing both recipient (grafted) and donor sites (Knighton 2020).

Advances in Wound Management Strategies for the Prevention of Hypertrophic Scarring

Biosynthetic skin substitutes are frequently employed for full-thickness burns, particularly those located on the extremities. A biodegradable temporizing matrix (BTM), comprising a wound-facing biodegradable polymer foam and a nonbiodegradable transparent sealing membrane, is typically applied to the full-thickness burn wound after surgical debridement for a minimum of 3 weeks (Frost et al. 2022). This facilitates wound granulation, neovascularization, and neo-dermis formation.

Closing monitoring is essential during neo-dermis formation. Accumulation of yellowish exudate or discharge beneath the BTM requires aspiration and draining to facilitate neo-dermis development (Dye 2021). Confirmation of the absence of infection is crucial. The BTM dressing should be inspected daily. Once adequate neovascularization and neo-dermis formation have occurred, the wound is closed surgically with a thin split-thickness skin graft.

A dermal regeneration template, such as Nevelia®, is occasionally employed for deep or full-thickness burn wounds (Hosseini and Shafiee 2021; De Angelis et al. 2018). Nevelia® consists of a wound-facing layer of stabilized type I bovine collagen and a reinforced silicone layer. Applied to the excised full-thickness burn wound for a minimum of 3 weeks, it facilitates cellular infiltration and subsequent tissue regeneration. Following this period, a thin split-thickness skin graft is typically applied.

The application of biosynthetic skin substitutes or dermal regeneration templates to deep partial-thickness or full-thickness burn wounds can mitigate hypertrophic scarring and contracture formation, thereby improving the quality of life for burn patients (Wong et al. 2023).

Pain Management

Pain management is a critical concern for burn patients, encompassing procedural, breakthrough, and background pain (Nosanov et al. 2020). Inadequate pain control can result in psychological distress and contribute to adverse physiological consequences, including hemodynamic instability and impaired wound healing. For conscious adult burn patients undergoing wound dressing changes, which are typically associated with severe pain, oral administration of a strong opioid, such as morphine syrup (0.3–0.5 mg/kg), is recommended 40 min prior to the procedure (Friedrichsdorf 2019; Klifto and Hultman 2024).

During wound dressing changes, pain assessment is essential. For adult burn patients, the Numeric Rating Scale, a self-report measure providing a subjective indication of pain intensity, can be utilized (Mahar et al. 2012). For pediatric burn patients, the Faces Pain Scale—Revised (FPS-R) is a suitable assessment tool (Shahi et al. 2020). The facial expressions depicted on the FPS-R correspond to different levels of pain intensity. Evaluation of pain response is necessary to monitor the effectiveness of analgesics. The impact of pain on the patient should also be assessed, including factors such as sleep disturbance, mood instability, and limitations in daily activities resulting from inadequate pain control. Consultation with the pain management team is recommended for prescribing appropriate targeted analgesics.

Multidisciplinary Team Approaches Enhance Optimizing Burn Patient Outcomes

Physiotherapy for Rehabilitation Support

Major burn injuries frequently involve soft tissue damage, which can lead to joint contractures. The optimal approach to managing joint contractures is preventive. This includes early initiation of active range-of-motion (ROM) exercises, restoration of joint range, and mobility training during acute care, along with appropriate surgical intervention for wound closure (Cartotto et al. 2023).

Upon admission, burn patients are prescribed active and passive mobilization and strengthening exercise tailored to the severity of their injuries. Progress is documented for ongoing evaluation. These exercises focus on maintaining full limb extension and flexion, as well as maintaining sustained strength.

The principle of progressive overload holds that a physiological system must be challenged at a level beyond its current capacity to elicit a training effect (American College of Sports Medicine 2013). This system gradually adapts to the imposed overload. Typical overload variables include intensity, duration, and frequency (sessions per week) of exercise. Increased strength facilitates force production, while enhanced muscular endurance improves sustained effort. Burn patients require muscle strengthening and resistance training to regain the ability to perform activities of daily living. Furthermore, burn patients engage in core and assistance exercise program (Rivas et al. 2020). Core exercises recruit one or more large muscle groups (e.g., chest, shoulders, and back). Assistance exercises, conversely, recruit smaller muscle groups, such as the biceps, triceps, and calf muscles.

Occupational Therapy for Rehabilitation Support

Given the potential for joint contractures as a complication of burn injuries (Fanstone and Price 2024). Maintaining optimal patient positioning is fundamental to achieving the best functional outcomes in burn rehabilitation (Ahuja et al. 2016; Parry et al. 2011). Positioning programs are implemented upon admission and continued throughout the rehabilitation process. Positioning is implemented to counteract deforming forces without compromising function. Considerations include the patient's respiratory status, burn area, wound depth, and associated injuries, such as exposed tendons or joints, and fractures. Individualized positioning programs are monitored regularly and adjusted according to the patient's evolving medical status. The principle "the position of comfort is the position of deformity" is particularly relevant to patients with serious burn injuries (Procter 2010). Proper positioning can be maintained using pillows, splints, serial casting, cutout foam, and other assertive devices (Serghiou et al. 2018). These devices are employed to achieve optimal positioning of the entire body and counteract the deforming forces of scare contraction. Positioning strategies are used to influence soft-tissue length, thereby limiting the loss of ROM due to scar formation and contracture. The ultimate goal is to optimize functional outcomes during rehabilitation.

Hypertrophic scar formation is another potential complication (Finnerty et al. 2016). Deeper wounds and prolonged healing increase the risk of hypertrophic scarring. During wound healing, collagen fibers are deposited to cover the wound surface, forming an immature scar, which typically appears red, rigid, and raised (van Baar 2020). Hypertrophic scar can cause itchiness, disfigurement, and contractures (Edwards 2022). The Vancouver burn scar scale, developed by Sullivan et al. (1990), provides a subjective assessment of burn scar pigmentation, vascularity, bendability, and height (Putri et al. 2024; Sullivan et al. 1990).

Pressure therapy is not required for all scars. Burn wounds that heal within 7–14 days generally do not necessitate pressure therapy (Sharp et al. 2016). Wounds healing within 14–21 days should be closely monitored to determine the potential need for intervention (Markiewicz-Gospodarek et al. 2022). Wounds requiring more than 21 days to heal typically require pressure garments and padding (Cancio et al. 2017). Custom-made pressure garments are effective in reducing vascularity, minimizing scar formation, decreasing scar thickness and firmness, and preventing contractures that restrict joint ROM (Atiyeh et al. 2013). For optimal effectiveness, pressure garments should be worn continuously, day and night, and removed only for bathing and occasionally during exercise that impedes movement.

Dietitian for Nutritional Support

Nutrition support is essential for optimizing the nutritional status of patients with severe burns by providing required nutrients and adjunctive therapeutic (Natarajan 2019). The goal is to meet the unique metabolic demands hypermetabolism, a state which can lead to life-threatening protein-calorie malnutrition in burn patients (Clark et al. 2017; Song et al. 2020).

Registered dietitians are consulted to develop and implement individualized nutritional management plans. These plans encompass the patient's prescribed diet, including necessary supplementation. Enteral nutritional support is administered via the oral route, or through nasogastric tube, gastric, or intestinal tubes as clinically indicated (Sudenis et al. 2015). Parenteral nutritional support is administered intravenously. Typically, parenteral nutrition is reserved for patients in whom enteral feeding is contraindicated or not tolerated. Early initiation of nutritional support, whether enteral or parenteral, is crucial in burn patients to prevent protein loss, eliminate infection rates, and minimize caloric deficits (Song et al. 2020; Peck et al. 2004). Furthermore, early initiation of enteral nutrition can improve gastrointestinal function, reduce ischemia-reperfusion injury, and decrease intestinal permeability in burn patients compared to those receiving parenteral nutrition (Clark et al. 2017). Adequate nutritional support is evidenced by increases in lean body mass and overall body weight (Badawy and Allam 2021; Hampton et al. 2021; Prins 2009).

Clinical Psychology-Psychosocial Support, Reintegration into Society, Fulfilling Life

Burn patients frequently encounter a range of psychosocial challenges during their recovery from severe burn injuries (Van Loey and Van Son 2003; Wong et al. 2023). These challenges encompass adapting to physical limitations and permanent alteration in appearance and function, coping with grief and loss, and managing the psychosocial impact of trauma. This impact can manifest as acute stress, anxiety, chronic pain, sleep disturbances, depression, and concerns regarding body image (Akarsu et al. 2017; Rosenberg et al. 2018; Van Loey and Van Son 2003). Furthermore, patients often face broader adjustment issues related to their altered life circumstances. Studies indicate that approximately 30% of burn survivors experience persistent psychosocial difficulties (Malt and Ugland 1989; Rosenberg et al. 2018).

Acute stress disorder (ASD) is characterized by the manifestation of acute stress reactions within the first month following a burn injury (Hobbs 2015; Smith et al. 2021; McKibben et al. 2008). The diagnostic criteria for ASD encompass symptoms clustered into five categories: intrusion, dissociation, negative mood, avoidance, and arousal (Bryant 2018; Geoffrion et al. 2022).

Post-traumatic stress disorder (PTSD) is a mental health disorder that can develop following a psychologically traumatic event, such as a severe burn injury (Lodha et al. 2020). Characteristics symptoms include intrusive thoughts, feelings, or dreams related to the traumatic event; psychological and physiological distress upon exposure to cues reminiscent of the trauma; negative alterations in cognition and mood; and heightened arousal, often manifested as an exaggerated fight-or-flight response (Brown 2017; Sommerhalder et al. 2020). These symptoms persist for more than 1 month after the traumatic event (Kornhaber et al. 2016).

Clinical psychologists are consulted to address the psychological needs of burn patients, including the assessment and treatment of conditions such as ASD and PTSD (McLean et al. 2017). Psychiatrists, rather than psychologists, are consulted for medication management (Griggs et al. 2017). Evidence-based stress-coping interventions, such as cognitive behavioral therapy, can be employed to mitigate patient stress and address related psychological needs (Dalal et al. 2010).

Conclusion

Comprehensive burn care requires integrated physical and psychosocial support. Nurses facilitate healing by fostering open communication and providing emotional support to patients and families. Ongoing physiotherapy and occupational therapy are essential for maximizing functional recovery and society reintegration.

References

Ahuja RB, Gibran N, Greenhalgh D, Jeng J, Mackie D, Moghazy A, Moiemen N, Palmieri T, Peck M, Serghiou M, Watson S, Wilson Y, ISBI Practice Guidelines Committee (2016) ISBI practice guidelines for burn care. Burns 42(5):953–1021. https://doi.org/10.1016/j.burns.2016.05.013

Akarsu S, Durmus M, Yapici AK, Oznur T, Ozturk S (2017) Psychiatric assessment and rehabilitation of burn patients. Turkish J Plast Surg 25(1):20–28. https://link.gale.com/apps/doc/A508361146/AONE?u=anon~cde7d1da&sid=googleScholar&xid=7affc17d. Accessed on 30 Oct 2024

American College of Sports Medicine (2013) ACSM'S guidelines for exercise testing and prescription. Lippincott Williams & Wilkins. https://books.google.com.hk/books?hl=zh-TW&lr=&id=hhosAwAAQBAJ&oi=fnd&pg=PP1&dq=Franklin+BA.+(2006)+General+principles+of+exercise+prescription.+ACSM%27s+Guidelines+for+Exercise+Testing+and+Prescription.+Lippincott+Williams+%26+Wilkins:+Philadelphia.&ots=llCb4IXVPA&sig=8Ew97yHY9vDvjvWjcR1655W4Inc&redir_esc=y#v=onepage&q&f=false. Accessed on 30 Oct 2024

Atiyeh BS, El Khatib AM, Dibo SA (2013) Pressure garment therapy (PGT) of burn scars: evidence-based efficacy. Ann Burns Fire Disasters 26(4):205. https://pmc.ncbi.nlm.nih.gov/articles/PMC3978593/. Accessed on 30 Oct 2024

Badawy MM, Allam NM (2021) Impact of adding protein supplementation to exercise training on lean body mass and muscle strength in burn patients. J Burn Care Res 42(5):968–974. https://doi.org/10.1093/jbcr/irab007

Brown A (2017) Post traumatic stress disorder (PTSD) awareness. Page Publishing Inc, La Vergne

Bryant RA (2018) The current evidence for acute stress disorder. Curr Psychiatry Rep 20:1–8. https://doi.org/10.1016/j.jpsychires.2011.10.007

Burgess JD, Watt KA, Kimble RM, Cameron CM (2019) Knowledge of childhood burn risks and burn first aid: cool runnings. Inj Prev 25(4):301–306. https://doi.org/10.1136/injuryprev-2017-042650

Burke-Smith A, Collier J, Jones I (2015) A comparison of non-invasive imaging modalities: infrared thermography, spectrophotometric intracutaneous analysis and laser Doppler imaging for the assessment of adult burns. Burns 41(8):1695–1707. https://doi.org/10.1016/j.burns.2015.06.023

Cancio LC, Barillo DJ, Kearns RD, Holmes JH IV, Conlon KM, Matherly AF, Cairns BA, Hickerson WL, Palmieri T (2017) Guidelines for burn care under austere conditions: surgical and nonsurgical wound management. J Burn Care Res 38(4):203–214. https://doi.org/10.1097/BCR.0000000000000368

Cartotto R, Johnson L, Rood JM, Lorello D, Matherly A, Parry I, Romanowski K, Wiechman S, Bettencourt A, Carson JS, Lam HT, Nedelec B (2023) Clinical practice guideline: early mobilization and rehabilitation of critically ill burn patients. J Burn Care Res 44(1):1–15. https://doi.org/10.1093/jbcr/irac008

Clark A, Imran J, Madni T, Wolf SE (2017) Nutrition and metabolism in burn patients. Burns Trauma 5(11):1–12. https://doi.org/10.1186/s41038-017-0076-x

Dalal PK, Saha R, Agarwal M (2010) Psychiatric aspects of burn. Indian J Plast Surg 43(S 01):S136–S142. https://doi.org/10.1055/s-0039-1699471

De Angelis B, Orlandi F, Fernandes Lopes Morais D'Autilio M, Scioli MG, Orlandi A, Cervelli V, Gentile P (2018) Long-term follow-up comparison of two different bi-layer dermal substitutes in tissue regeneration: clinical outcomes and histological findings. Int Wound J 15(5):695–706. https://doi.org/10.1111/iwj.12912

Dye JF (2021) From secondary intent to accelerated regenerative healing: emergence of the bio-intelligent scaffold vasculogenic strategy for skin reconstruction. In: Vascularization for tissue engineering and regenerative medicine, pp 205–271. https://doi.org/10.1007/978-3-319-54586-8_20

Edwards J (2022) Hypertrophic scar management. Br J Nurs 31(20):S24–S31. https://doi.org/10.12968/bjon.2022.31.20.S24

Esin S, Kaya E, Maisetta G, Romanelli M, Batoni G (2022) The antibacterial and antibiofilm activity of Granudacyn in vitro in a 3D collagen wound infection model. J Wound Care 31(11):908–922. https://doi.org/10.12968/jowc.2022.31.11.908

Fanstone R, Price P (2024) Global perspectives on risk factors for major joint burn contractures: a literature review. Burns 50(3):537–549. https://doi.org/10.1016/j.burns.2023.09.014

Finnerty CC, Jeschke MG, Branski LK, Barret JP, Dziewulski P, Herndon DN (2016) Hypertrophic scarring: the greatest unmet challenge after burn injury. Lancet 388(10052):1427–1436. https://doi.org/10.1016/S0140-6736(16)31406-4

Friedrichsdorf SJ (2019) Treatment and prevention of pain in children and adults. In: Handbook of burns volume 1: acute burn care, p 323. https://doi.org/10.1007/978-3-030-18940-2_25

Frost SR, Deodhar A, Offer GJ (2022) A novel use for the biodegradable temporizing matrix. Eur J Plast Surg 45(6):1015–1020. https://doi.org/10.1007/s00238-022-01964-z

Geoffrion S, Goncalves J, Robichaud I, Sader J, Giguere CE, Fortin M, Lamothe J, Bernard P, Guay S (2022) Systematic review and meta-analysis on acute stress disorder: rates following different types of traumatic events. Trauma Violence Abuse 23(1):213–223. https://doi.org/10.1177/1524838020933844

Gill P (2013) The critical evaluation of laser doppler imaging in determining burn depth. Int J Burns Trauma 3(2):72–77

Gillies A (2019) Surfactants in the treatment of chronic wounds and biofilm management. J Community Nurs 33(6):34–38

Giretzlehner M, Ganitzer I, Haller H (2021) Technical and medical aspects of burn size assessment and documentation. Medicina 57(3):242. https://doi.org/10.3390/medicina57030242

Griggs C, Goverman J, Bittner E, Levi B (2017) Sedation and pain management in burn patients. Clin Plast Surg 44(3):535. https://doi.org/10.1015/j.cps.2017.02.026

Hampton V, Hampton T, Dheansa B, Falder S, Emery P (2021) Evaluation of high protein intake to improve clinical outcome and nutritional status for patients with burns: a systematic review. Burns 47(8):1714–1729. https://doi.org/10.1016/j.burns.2021.02.028

Harish V, Tiwari N, Fisher OM, Li Z, Maitz PK (2019) First aid improves clinical outcomes in burn injuries: evidence from a cohort study of 4918 patients. Burns 45(2):433–439. https://doi.org/10.1016/j.burns.2018.09.024

Hobbs K (2015) Which factors influence the development of post-traumatic stress disorder in patients with burn injuries? A systematic review of the literature. Burns 41(3):421–430. https://doi.org/10.1016/j.burns.2014.10.018

Hosseini M, Shafiee A (2021) Engineering bioactive scaffolds for skin regeneration. Small 17(41):2101384. https://doi.org/10.1002/smll.202101384

Jonsson A, Bonander C, Nilson F, Huss F (2017) The state of the residential fire fatality problem in Sweden: epidemiology, risk factors, and event typologies. J Saf Res 62:89–100. https://doi.org/10.1016/j.jsr.2017.06.008

Klifto KM, Hultman CS (2024) Pain management in burn patients: pharmacologic management of acute and chronic pain. Clin Plast Surg 51(2):267–301. https://doi.org/10.1016/j.cps.2023.11.004

Knighton J (2020) Nursing management of the burn patient. In: Handbook of burns volume 1: acute burn care, pp 347–384. https://doi.org/10.1007/978-3-030-18940-2_27

Kornhaber R, Bridgman H, McLean L, & Vandervord J (2016). The role of resilience in the recovery of the burn-injured patient: an integrative review. Chronic Wound Care Management and Research, 41–50. https://doi.org/10.2147/CWCMR.S94618

Kotecha VR, Opot NE, Nangole F (2022) Assessment and management of pain in patients sustaining burns at emergency department Kenyatta National Hospital, Kenya: a descriptive study. Trauma Care 2(1):79–86. https://doi.org/10.3390/traumacare2010007

Lodha P, Shah B, Karia S, De Sousa A (2020) Post-traumatic stress disorder (PTSD) following burn injuries: a comprehensive clinical review. Ann Burns Fire Disasters 33(4):276. https://pmc.ncbi.nlm.nih.gov/articles/PMC7894845/. Accessed on 30 Oct 2024

Mahar PD, Wasiak J, O'Loughlin CJ, Christelis N, Arnold CA, Spinks AB, Danilla S (2012) Frequency and use of pain assessment tools implemented in randomized controlled trials in the adult burns population: a systematic review. Burns 38(2):147–154. https://doi.org/10.1016/j.burns.2011.09.015

Malt UF, Ugland OM (1989) A long-term psychosocial follow-up study of burned adults. Acta Psychiatr Scand 80:94–102. https://doi.org/10.1111/j.1600-0447.1989.tb05259.x

Markiewicz-Gospodarek A, Kozioł M, Tobiasz M, Baj J, Radzikowska-Büchner E, Przekora A (2022) Burn wound healing: clinical complications, medical care, treatment, and dressing types: the current state of knowledge for clinical practice. Int J Environ Res Public Health 19(3):1338. https://doi.org/10.3390/ijerph19031338

Mayer DO, Tettelbach WH, Ciprandi G, Downie F, Hampton J, Hodgson H, Lazaro-Martinez JL, Probst A, Schultz G, Stürmer EK, Parnham A, Frescos N, Stand D, Holloway S, Percival SL (2024) Best practice for wound debridement. J Wound Care 33(Sup6b):S1–S32. https://doi.org/10.12968/jowc.2024.33.Sup6b.S1

McKibben JB, Bresnick MG, Wiechman Askay SA, Fauerbach JA (2008) Acute stress disorder and posttraumatic stress disorder: A prospective study of prevalence, course, and predictors in a sample with major burn injuries. J Burn Care Res 29(1):22–35. https://doi.org/10.1097/BCR.0b013e31815f59c4

McLean L, Chen R, Kwiet J, Streimer J, Vandervord J, Kornhaber R (2017) A clinical update on posttraumatic stress disorder in burn injury survivors. Australas Psychiatry 25(4):348–350. https://doi.org/10.1177/1039856217700285

McLure M, Macneil F, Wood FM, Cuttle L, Eastwood K, Bray J, Tracy LM (2021) A rapid review of burns first aid guidelines: is there consistency across international guidelines? Cureus 13(6). https://doi.org/10.7759/cureus.15779

Natarajan M (2019) Recent concepts in nutritional therapy in critically ill burn patients. Int J Nutr Pharmacol Neurol Dis 9(1):4–36. https://doi.org/10.4103/ijnpnd.ijnpnd_58_18

Nosanov LB, Brandt JL, Schneider DM, Johnson LS (2020) Pain management in burn patients. Curr Trauma Rep 6:161–173. https://doi.org/10.1007/s40719-020-00203-9

Parry I, Esselman PC, Rehabilitation Committee of the American Burn Association (2011) Clinical competencies for burn rehabilitation therapists. J Burn Care Res 32(4):458–467. https://doi.org/10.1097/BCR.0b013e318220c15a

Peck MD, Kessler M, Cairns BA, Chang YH, Ivanova A, Schooler W (2004) Early enteral nutrition does not decrease hypermetabolism associated with burn injury. J Trauma Acute Care Surg 57(6):1143–1149. https://doi.org/10.1097/01.TA.0000145826.84657.38

Prins A (2009) Nutritional management of the burn patient. S Afr J Clin Nutr 22(1):9–15. https://doi.org/10.10520/EJC65058

Procter F (2010) Rehabilitation of the burn patient. Indian J Plast Surg 43(Suppl):S101. https://doi.org/10.4103/0970-0358.70730

Putri IL, Sindhu FC, Aisyah IF, Pramanasari R, Wungu CDK (2024) Comparison of combination skin substitutes and skin grafts versus skin grafts only for treating wounds measured by Vancouver scar scale: a comprehensive meta-analysis. SAGE Open Med 12:20503121241266342. https://doi.org/10.1177/20503121241266342

Rivas E, McEntire SJ, Kowalske KJ, Suman OE (2020) Exercise. In: Handbook of burns volume 2: reconstruction and rehabilitation, p 125. https://doi.org/10.1007/978-3-030-34511-2_13

Rosenberg L, Rosenberg M, Rimmer RB, Fauerbach JA (2018) Psychosocial recovery and reintegration of patients with burn injuries. In: Total burn care. Elsevier, pp 709–720. https://doi.org/10.1016/B978-0-323-47661-4.00065-4

Rossella E, Giulio M, Michele M (2022) Burns: classification and treatment. In: Maruccia M, Giudice G (eds) Textbook of plastic and reconstructive surgery: basic principles and new perspectives. Springer, Cham, pp 285–301. https://doi.org/10.1007/978-3-030-82335-1_18

Salehi SH, Momeni M, Vahdani M, Moradi M (2020) Clinical value of debriding enzymes as an adjunct to standard early surgical excision in human burns: a systematic review. J Burn Care Res 41(6):1224–1230. https://doi.org/10.1093/jbcr/iraa074

Serghiou MA, Ott S, Cowan A, Kemp-Offenberg J, Suman OE (2018) Burn rehabilitation along the continuum of care. In: Total burn care. Elsevier, pp 476–508. https://doi.org/10.1016/B978-0-323-47661-4.00046-0

Shahi N, Meier M, Phillips R, Shirek G, Goldsmith A, Recicar J, Zuk J, Bielsky A, Yaster M, Moulton S (2020) Pain management for pediatric burns in the outpatient setting: A changing paradigm? J Burn Care Res 41(4):814–819. https://doi.org/10.1093/jbcr/iraa049

Sharp PA, Pan B, Yakuboff KP, Rothchild D (2016) Development of a best evidence statement for the use of pressure therapy for management of hypertrophic scarring. J Burn Care Res 37(4):255–264. https://doi.org/10.1097/BCR.0000000000000253

Smith MB, Wiechman SA, Mandell SP, Gibran NS, Vavilala MS, Rivara FP (2021) Current practices and beliefs regarding screening patients with burns for acute stress disorder and post-traumatic stress disorder: A survey of the American burn association membership. Eur Burn J 2(4):215–225. https://doi.org/10.3390/ebj2040016

Sommerhalder C, Blears E, Murton AJ, Porter C, Finnerty C, Herndon DN (2020) Current problems in burn hypermetabolism. Curr Probl Surg 57(1):100709. https://doi.org/10.1016/j.cpsurg.2019.100709

Song J, Wolf SE, Wade CE, Ziegler TR (2020) Specialized nutrition support in burns, wasting, deconditioning, and hypermetabolic conditions. In: Present knowledge in nutrition. Academic, pp 619–636. https://doi.org/10.1016/B978-0-12-818460-8.00034-4

Sudenis T, Hall K, Cartotto R (2015) Enteral nutrition: what the dietitian prescribes is not what the burn patient gets! J Burn Care Res 36(2):297–305. https://doi.org/10.1097/BCR.0000000000000069

Sullivan TA, Smith J, Kermode J, McIver E, Courtemanche DJ (1990) Rating the burn scar. J Burn Care Rehabil 11(3):256–260. https://doi.org/10.1097/00004630-199005000-00014

van Baar ME (2020) Epidemiology of scars and their consequences: burn scars. In: Textbook on scar management: state of the art management and emerging technologies, pp 37–43. https://doi.org/10.1007/978-3-030-44766-3_5

Van Loey NE, Van Son MJ (2003) Psychopathology and psychological problems in patients with burn scars: epidemiology and management. Am J Clin Dermatol 4:245–272. https://doi.org/10.2165/00128071-200304040-00004

Wang R, Zhao J, Zhang Z, Cao C, Zhang Y, Mao Y (2020) Diagnostic accuracy of laser doppler imaging for the assessment of burn depth: a meta-analysis and systematic review. J Burn Care Res 41(3):619–625. https://doi.org/10.1093/jbcr/irz203

Wong TW, Yip KH, Yip YC, Tsui WK (2023) Advances in burn care in Hong Kong: reflecting on a decade of expert experiences from local practice with an international perspective. In: New research in nursing-education and practice. IntechOpen. https://doi.org/10.5772/intechopen.110319

Zou K, Wynn PM, Miller P, Hindmarch P, Majsak-Newman G, Young B, Hayer M, Kendrick D (2015) Preventing childhood scalds within the home: overview of systematic reviews and a systematic review of primary studies. Burns 41(5):907–924. https://doi.org/10.1016/j.burns.2014.11.002

Advancements in Chest Drainage Systems for Cardiothoracic Surgery Patients

13

Oi-Lin Wut and Alice Yip

Introduction

Thoracic surgical procedures that comprise the pleural membrane may result in the accumulation of fluid (pleural effusion) or air (pneumothorax) within the pleural cavity (Williams and Lerner 2021). This accumulation can disrupt the negative intrapleural pressure required for effective pulmonary expansion. Chest tube insertion facilitates the evacuation of fluid or air from the pleural space, thereby restoring negative intrapleural pressure and promoting optimal pulmonary function (Nakada and Ohtsuka 2023; Walcott-Sapp and Sukumar 2015).

The maintenance of a patent chest drainage system is essential for alleviating postoperative complications in cardiothoracic surgery (Gao et al. 2019; St-Onge et al. 2021.) Compromised pleural drainage can lead to complications, including respiratory insufficiency, infection, and progressive pulmonary collapse (Luyt et al. 2020; Matthay et al. 2019). Chest drainage reduces these risks by maintaining pleural space patency (Lobdell and Engelman 2023). Furthermore, it promotes postoperative recovery by facilitating adequate ventilation and optimizing gas exchange. Studies have shown that effective drainage can lead to diminishing postoperative pain and shorter hospital stays, as it allows for better lung function and mobility (Kim 2023; Li et al. 2019). Conversely, poor drainage can cause breathing problems and a longer recovery time (Anderson et al. 2022).

O.-L. Wut (✉)
Hong Kong College of Surgical Nursing, Kowloon, HKSAR, China
e-mail: wutoilin@ha.org.hk

A. Yip
School of Health Sciences, St. Francis University,
Tseung Kwan O, Hong Kong
e-mail: khyip@sfu.edu.hk

Three centuries of chest drainage evolution have yielded substantial improvements in patient outcomes, facilitated reductions in the length of hospital stay, and elevated the overall standard of care (Bedawi et al. 2021; Foley and Parrish 2023; Lobdell and Engelman 2023).

Mechanism of Respiration

A comprehensive understanding of respiratory mechanics is essential for healthcare professionals, particularly in the context of managing patients utilizing thoracic drainage systems, including the three-chamber apparatus (Bawaadam et al. 2022). The fundamental physiological role of the respiratory system is to mediate the exchange of gases. A thorough understanding of the mechanisms governing pulmonary expansion and contraction is critical for the evaluation of respiratory function and the identification of potential complications associated with thoracic drainage systems, including pneumothorax or pleural effusion. An understanding of respiratory physiology highlights the significance of negative intrapleural pressure, a critical factor in comprehending the mechanism by which a chest tube facilitates the restoration of pulmonary function (Sorino et al. 2024).

Pulmonary ventilation, a complex physiological process encompassing the two-way movement of air into and out of the lungs, is fundamentally predicated on the principles of negative intrapleural pressure. This negative pressure is essential for pulmonary expansion and regulates airflow during both inspiratory and expiratory phases. A comprehensive understanding of these mechanics, including their clinical implications, enables healthcare professionals, such as nurses, to effectively manage respiratory pathologies and optimize ventilatory support strategies.

The cyclical volume changes within the thoracic cavity, arranged by the diaphragm and intercostal muscles, drive pulmonary ventilation. During inspiration, their contraction expands the thoracic cavity, decreasing intrapleural pressure and drawing air into the lungs. Conversely, during expiration, the relaxation of these muscles reduces thoracic cavity volume, increasing intrapleural pressure and expelling air from the lungs (Betts et al. 2022). The interchange of muscle action and pressure dynamics forms the basis of respiration.

Historical Background

The application of chest tubes in medical practice dates to the eighteenth century, initially employed for the evacuation of blood in cases of traumatic hemothorax. Closed drainage systems emerged in the late nineteenth century, notably with Gotthard Bülau's introduction of a water-sealed system in 1875 (Lobdell et al. 2024). This innovation revolutionized the management of pleural effusions, including empyema (characterized by the accumulation of pus within the pleural space), by facilitating effective drainage, maintaining negative intrapleural pressure, preventing air reentry, and, thereby, alleviating symptoms and improving patient outcomes.

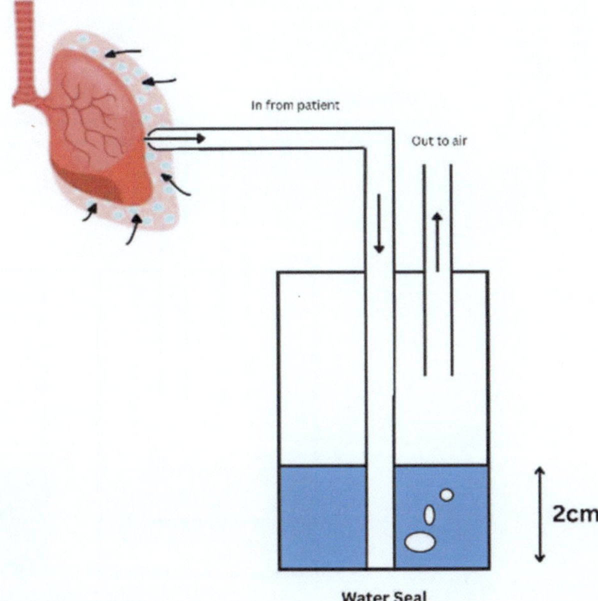

Fig. 13.1 The diagram of a one-bottle drainage system

One-Bottle Chest Drainage System

The one-bottle drainage system design facilitated ease of implementation and management for healthcare providers (Sorino et al. 2024). A closed-water-seal mechanism ensured continuous drainage of air and fluid while preventing reentry of air into the pleural cavity. This was crucial for maintaining negative intrapleural pressure, thereby promoting lung expansion and improved respiratory function. The system's one-bottle design streamlined setup and management, with the collection bottle serving dually as a fluid reservoir and a water seal to prevent backflow (Fig. 13.1).

Two-Bottle Chest Drainage System

The two-bottle system comprises a collection chamber and a water-seal chamber (Fig. 13.2) (Sorino et al. 2024). The patient-proximal collection chamber accumulates pleural fluid and air, enabling precise volumetric measurement crucial for patient monitoring. Distal to the collection chamber, the water chamber, the water-seal chamber functions as a unidirectional valve, facilitating air exit while precluding reentry into the pleural space. This is achieved via a water column (typically 2 cm), which acts as a one-way valve, permitting air expulsion during exhalation and preventing access during inhalation (Anderson et al. 2022; Zisis et al. 2015).

The two-bottle chest drainage system utilizes gravity and respiratory mechanics to effect drainage (Sorino et al. 2024). Exhalation propels air and fluid from the

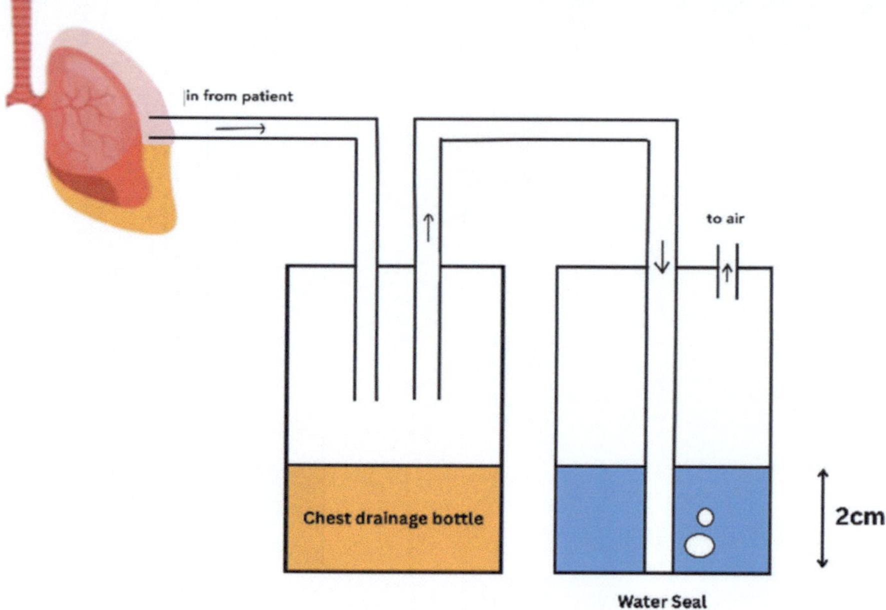

Fig. 13.2 The diagram of a two-bottle drainage system

pleural cavity into the collection chamber. The water seal maintains negative intrapleural pressure, essential for lung re-expansion and pneumothorax prevention. Continuous monitoring of fluid output and air leaks is facilitated by observation of water column fluctuations reflecting intrathoracic pressure changes during respiration. Compared to more complex systems, its compact design enhances manageability. The inherent water-seal mechanism effectively prevents air reentry into the pleural space (Anderson et al. 2022; Zisis et al. 2015). Its cost-effectiveness makes it suitable for resource-constrained settings. However, accumulating fluid may impede drainage, necessitating frequent monitoring, and the absence of regulated suction may limit efficacy in specific clinical scenarios.

Three-Bottle Chest Drainage System

Several chest drainage system designs have evolved overtime. While one- and two-bottle systems exist, the three-bottle system, introduced at Massachusetts General Hospital in 1945, established itself as a standard for managing pleural effusions and air leaks (Fig. 13.3) (George and Papagiannopoulos 2016; Sorino et al. 2024; Zisis et al. 2015). Similar to the two-bottle system, it incorporates collection and water-seal chambers; however, a third chamber provides suction control. This chamber connects to the water-seal chamber, enabling adjustable negative pressure application to enhance drainage. The controlled suction facilitates more rapid evacuation of

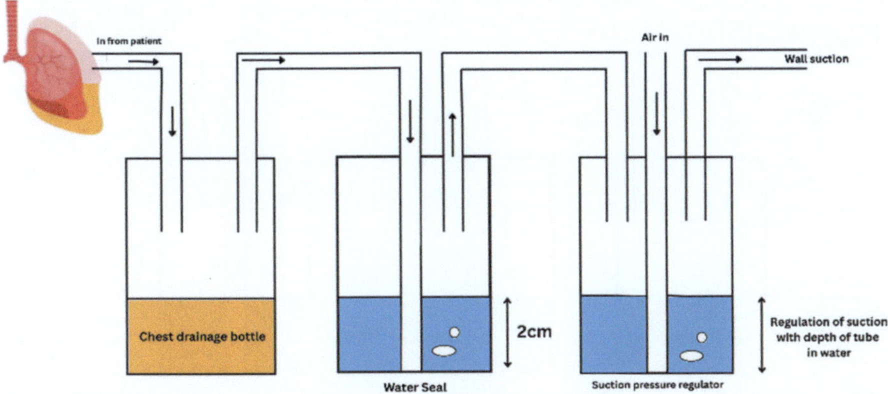

Fig. 13.3 The diagram of a three-bottle drainage system

air and fluid from the pleural space, proving particularly beneficial in cases of substantial air leaks or significant fluid accumulation (Zisis et al. 2015).

The three-bottle system allows for simultaneous monitoring of fluid drainage and air leaks indicated by bubbling in the water-seal chamber (George and Papagiannopoulos 2016; Sorino et al. 2024). Its enhanced drainage capacity, achieved through controlled suction, makes it preferable in cases requiring rapid removal of significant air or fluid, such as in hemothorax or large pneumothorax (Anderson et al. 2022). However, its increased bulk and potential for accidental disconnections or blockages, compared to the two-bottle system, may present challenges in resource-limited environments (Anderson et al. 2022; Zisis et al. 2015). Both two- and three-bottle systems are valuable in managing pleural conditions; the two-bottle system's simplicity and cost-effectiveness suit uncomplicated cases, while the three-bottle system's superior drainage capabilities, facilitated by suction control, are advantageous in more complex clinical presentations.

The conventional three-bottle chest drainage system often restricts patient mobility, contributing to discomfort and potentially prolonged hospital stays (Sorino et al. 2024). Subjective assessment of air leaks inherent in traditional systems can lead to inconsistent clinical decision-making. Furthermore, the complexity of older design increases the risk of infection due to the multiplicity of connections and the potential for disconnections.

Disposable Integrated Chest-Drainage Box (Three-Bottle System)

Modern clinical practice predominantly utilizes integrated chest drainage units, representing an evolution from the traditional three-bottle system (Sorino et al. 2024). While Deknatel's introduction of the first disposable unit predates current integrated systems in 1967, it marked a significant advancement (Sorino et al. 2024; Zisis et al. 2015). These integrated systems enhance the efficiency of pleural fluid and air

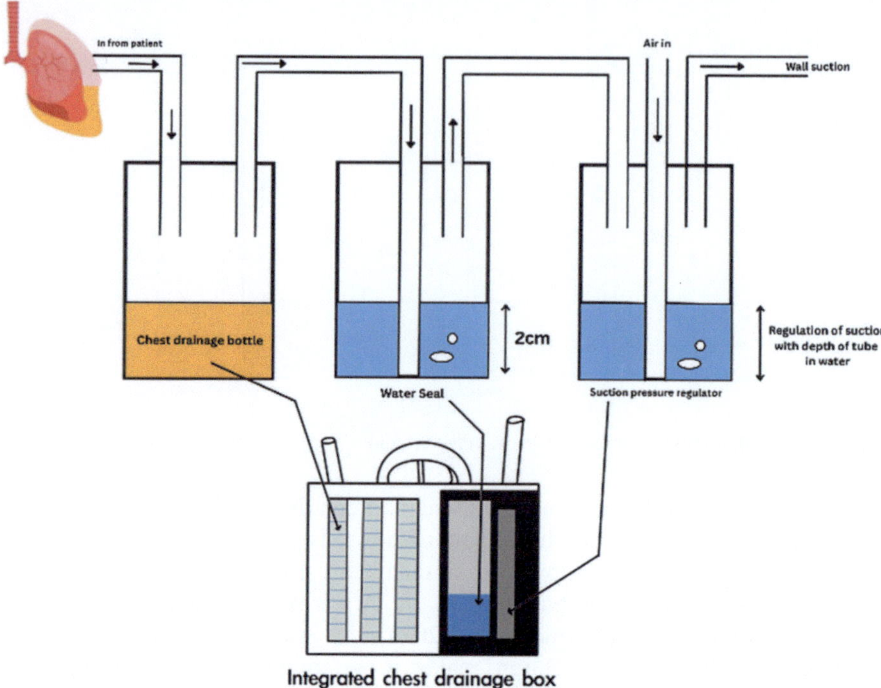

Fig. 13.4 Diagram of integrated chest drainage box

removal by incorporating collection, water-seal, and suction control chambers with a single, compact unit (Anderson et al. 2022; Zisis et al. 2015). The widespread adoption of disposable systems in the late twentieth century significantly improved hygiene and reduced infection risk, thereby enhancing both the safety and efficiency of chest drainage procedures (Wang et al. 2019). Following the introduction of the three-chamber system, numerous manufacturers developed and commercialized integrated chest drainage systems (Fig. 13.4).

The streamlined setup and operation of disposable integrated chest drainage systems offer healthcare professionals simplified chest drainage management. These systems substantially mitigate the risk of cross-contamination and infection compared to reusable alternatives. Eliminating the need for cleaning sterilization contributes to cost-effectiveness, making disposable systems economically advantageous over time. Furthermore, the inherent design facilitates visual monitoring of drainage output and air leaks while also enabling more convenient patient transport compared to traditional chest drainage systems (Anderson et al. 2022).

Improper utilization of integrated chest drainage systems can result in significant complications, including iatrogenic lung injury, such as tension pneumothorax, particularly through mismanagement of pressure within the water-seal chamber (Anderson et al. 2022). To mitigate the risk of excessive negative pressure

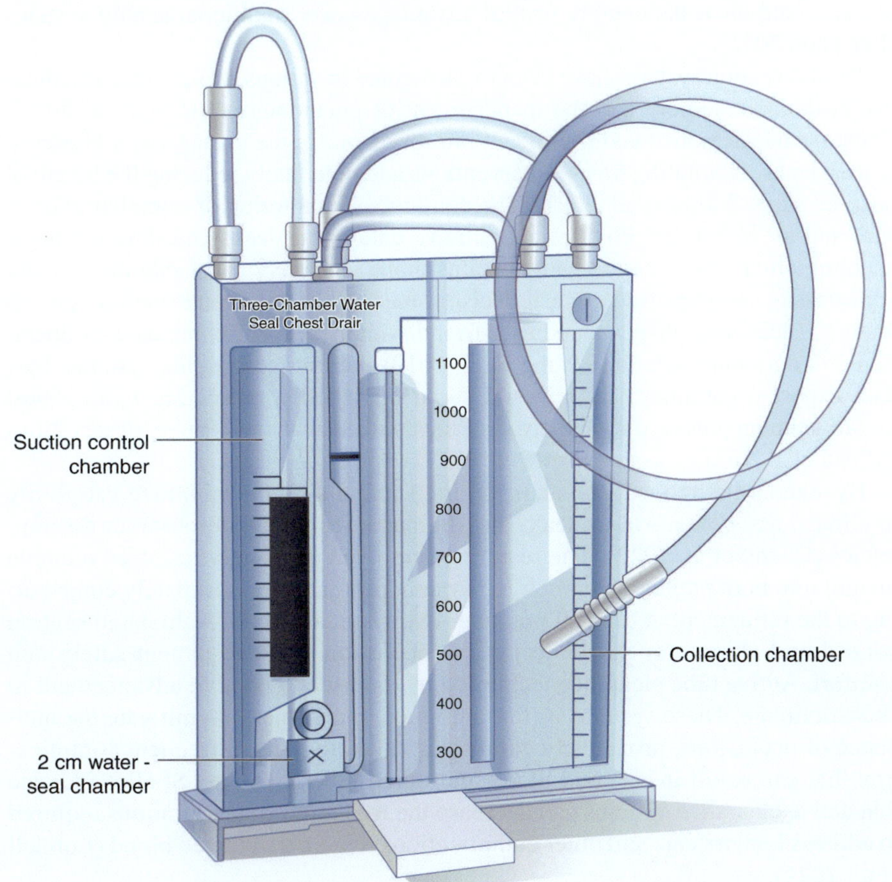

Fig. 13.5 Integrated chest drainage system

accumulation, manufacturers have incorporated a manual high negative pressure relief valve into these systems (Fig. 13.5). Proficiency in the proper operation of this system is crucial for all healthcare professionals involved in its use (Zisis et al. 2015).

Development of Digital Suction System

Digital suction systems represent a substantial advancement in medical technology for managing thoracic drainage (Lee et al. 2021). These systems offer enhanced monitoring and control capabilities compared to traditional suction methods. By providing real-time, objective measurements of air leaks and fluid drainage, they reduce interobserver variability and facilitate quantitative analysis, ultimately contributing to improved patient outcomes. Furthermore, the utilization of electronic sensors and digital interfaces for precise measurement and control of intrathoracic pressure and air leaks confers several advantages over traditional analog systems (Lee et al. 2021).

Digital suction systems have been implemented in various clinical settings, notably in thoracic surgery and the management of pneumothorax (Lee et al. 2021). Their use has demonstrated significant improvements in the management of persistent air leaks, facilitating timely interventions and potentially reducing the length of hospital stays (Mitsui et al. 2021). The continuous monitoring of intrapleural pressure and air leak rates provides quantitative data on air leaks and fluid drainage, enabling clinicians to assess patient status more accurately and facilitating timely adjustments and improved clinical decision-making. Many digital suction systems feature touchscreen displays and user-friendly interfaces, enriching ease of operation and data interpretation (Wang et al. 2019). Furthermore, some systems offer data export capabilities via universal serial bus (USB), promoting more robust record-keeping based on objective metrics rather than subjective observations (Mitsui et al. 2021).

By standardizing measurements, digital suction systems minimize variability in clinical assessments of air leaks and drainage, reducing interobserver discrepancies (Chang et al. 2022). The resulting improved data analytics offer valuable insight into both patient outcomes and system performance, ultimately contributing to the refinement of clinical practices (Mitsui et al. 2021). Automated suction control and alarms for disconnection or occlusion improve patient safety and comfort. Active tube clearance technologies represent a notable advancement in chest drainage. These systems utilize automatic mechanisms to mitigate the incidence of occlusions, proactively addressing tube clogging, a frequent complication that can result in retained blood and other adverse events. Studies indicate that active clearance systems can decrease the frequency of reoperations required to address hemorrhage and other complications related to retained blood (Lobdell et al. 2024).

Digital suction systems improve patient comfort during recovery through noise reduction and enhanced drainage efficiency (Lee et al. 2021). Increased patient mobility afforded by these systems can further promote recovery and potentially shorten hospital stays. Moreover, the quantitative data generated by digital systems aids clinicians in determining the optimal timing for chest tube removal, a crucial aspect of patient recovery (Mitsui et al. 2021).

Studies indicate that patients managed with digital suction systems may experience shorter hospital stays and fewer complications compared to those using traditional systems (Lee et al. 2021; Sorino et al. 2024; Zhou et al. 2023). This improved clinical outcome is supported by research demonstrating that digital systems significantly reduce chest drainage duration and length of stay. Randomized controlled trials have further shown a reduction in prolonged air leaks, which are associated with extended recovery times and increased healthcare costs (Collins et al. 1995; Sorino et al. 2024; Zhou et al. 2023). While the initial investment in digital systems may be higher, the potential for reduced hospital stays and complications can result in overall cost saving (Lee et al. 2021; Sorino et al. 2024).

Future Development

Continued technological advancement and integration will shape the future of chest drainage systems (Lobdell and Engelman 2023; Sorino et al. 2024). Key areas for development include remote patient monitoring and intervention through telemedicine. Additionally, artificial intelligence could enable personalized drainage protocols based on individual patient characteristics, optimizing recovery and outcomes.

Effective implementation and utilization of emerging technologies in chest drainage necessitate ongoing education and training for healthcare professionals, especially frontline nurses. Established Enhanced Recovery After Surgery (ERAS) guideline will influence the future development of chest drainage systems, promoting digital systems for improved decision-making and patient outcomes (ERAS® Society 2024). Discouraging routine external suction due to limited benefits and potential complications, the guidelines emphasize regular monitoring and maintenance of chest tube patency to prevent retained blood complications (ERAS® Society 2024; Piler et al. 2024).

Drainless techniques in thoracic surgery represent an important area of development (Liao et al. 2020; Lobdell et al. 2024). Their feasibility depends on the surgical procedure, patient condition, and specific clinical circumstances. Offering significant comfort and recovery benefits for select patients, these techniques will be further refined through ongoing research and clinical experience to establish best practices for individualized care.

Conclusion

From early one-bottle systems to the complexity of three-bottle setups, chest drainage has evolved significantly, driven by the persistent need to effectively manage air leaks and fluid accumulation, ultimately improving patient outcomes. This evolution, fostered by technological advancements, has led to digital suction systems guided by standardized protocols, like ERAS, and even explored drainless techniques. Further technological advancements promise continued refinement of chest drainage, offering hope for even better patient care and recovery in the future.

Acknowledgments We acknowledge the contribution of Wong Pui Chak Marcus, who provided dedicated support for the graphical elements in this chapter.

References

Anderson D, Chen SA, Godoy LA, Brown LM, Cooke DT (2022) Comprehensive review of chest tube management: a review. JAMA Surg 157(3):269–274. https://doi.org/10.1001/jamasurg.2021.7050

Bawaadam HS, Boberg M, Gesthalter YB (2022) Ambulatory management of a recurrent pneumothorax with an indwelling tunneled pleural catheter. J Bronchol Interv Pulmonol 29(2):e15–e18. https://doi.org/10.1097/LBR.0000000000000782

Bedawi EO, Guinde J, Rahman NM, Astoul P (2021) Advances in pleural infection and malignancy. Eur Respir Rev 30(159). https://doi.org/10.1183/16000617.0002-2020

Betts JG, Young KA, DeSaix P (2022) Smooth muscle. In: Anatomy and physiology, 2nd edn. OpenStax CNX, pp 932–940

Chang PC, Chen KH, Jhou HJ, Lee CH, Chou SH, Chen PH, Chang TW (2022) Promising effects of digital chest tube drainage system for pulmonary resection: a systematic review and network meta-analysis. J Pers Med 12(4):512. https://doi.org/10.3390/jpm12040512

Collins CD, Lopez A, Mathie A, Wood V, Jackson JE, Roddie ME (1995) Quantification of pneumothorax size on chest radiographs using interpleural distances: regression analysis based on volume measurements from helical CT. Am J Roentgenol 165(5):1127–1130. https://doi.org/10.2214/ajr.165.5.7572489

ERAS® Society (2024) Enhanced recovery after surgery guidelines for chest tube management. ERAS J. Available online: https://erassociety.org/guidelines/. Accessed on 20 July 2025

Foley SP, Parrish JS (2023) Pleural space infections. Life 13(2):376. https://doi.org/10.3390/life13020376

Gao S, Barello S, Chen L, Chen C, Che G, Cai K, Crisci R, D'Andrilli A, Droghetti A, Fu X, Ferrari PA, Fernando HC, Ge D, Graffigna G, Huang Y, Hu J, Jiao W, Jiang G, Li X, Li H, Li S, Liu L, Ma D, Martinez G, Maurizi G, Phan K, Qiao K, Refai M, Rendina EA, Shao G, Shen J, Tian H, Voltolini L, Vannucci J, Vanni C, Wu Q, Xu S, Yu F, Zhao S, Zhang P, Zhang L, Zhi X, Zhu C, Ng C, Sihoe A, Ho AM (2019) Clinical guidelines on perioperative management strategies for enhanced recovery after lung surgery. Transl Lung Cancer Res 8(6):1174. https://doi.org/10.21037/tlcr.2019.12.25

George RS, Papagiannopoulos K (2016) Advances in chest drain management in thoracic disease. J Thorac Dis 8(Suppl 1):S55. https://doi.org/10.3978/j.issn.2072-1439.2015.11.19

Kim MP (2023) Chest tubes are painful. Ann Thorac Surg 115(4):843–844. https://doi.org/10.1016/j.athoracsur.2022.05.006

Lee SA, Kim JS, Chee HK, Hwang JJ, Ji M, Kim YH, Moon HJ, Lee WS (2021) Clinical application of a digital thoracic drainage system for objectifying and quantifying air leak versus the traditional vacuum system: a retrospective observational study. J Thorac Dis 13(2):1020. https://doi.org/10.21037/jtd-20-2993

Li P, Li S, Che G (2019) Role of chest tube drainage in physical function after thoracoscopic lung resection. J Thorac Dis 11(Suppl 15):S1947. https://doi.org/10.21037/jtd.2019.08.26

Liao HC, Yang SM, Hung MH, Cheng YJ, Hsu HH, Chen JS (2020) Thoracoscopic surgery without drainage tube placement for peripheral lung nodules. Ann Thorac Surg 109(3):887–893. https://doi.org/10.1016/j.athoracsur.2019.10.048

Lobdell KW, Engelman DT (2023) Chest tube management: past, present, and future directions for developing evidence-based best practices. Innovations 18(1):41–48. https://doi.org/10.1177/15569845231153623

Lobdell KW, Perrault LP, Drgastin RH, Brunelli A, Cerfolio RJ, Engelman DT, ERAS Cardiac Society Working Group (2024) Drainology: leveraging research in chest-drain management to enhance recovery after cardiothoracic surgery. JTCVS Tech 25:226–240. https://doi.org/10.1016/j.xjtc.2024.04.001

Luyt CE, Bouadma L, Morris AC, Dhanani JA, Kollef M, Lipman J, Martin-Loeches I, Nseir S, Ranzani OT, Roquilly A, Schmidt M, Torres A, Timsit JF (2020) Pulmonary infections complicating ARDS. Intensive Care Med 46:2168–2183. https://doi.org/10.1007/s00134-020-06292-z

Matthay MA, Zemans RL, Zimmerman GA, Arabi YM, Beitler JR, Mercat A, Herridge M, Randolph AG, Calfee CS (2019) Acute respiratory distress syndrome. Nat Rev Dis Prim 5(1):18. https://doi.org/10.1038/s41572-019-0069-0

Mitsui S, Tauchi S, Uchida T, Ohnishi H, Shimokawa T, Tobe S (2021) Low suction on digital drainage devices promptly improves post-operative air leaks following lung resection operations: a retrospective study. J Cardiothorac Surg 16:1–7. https://doi.org/10.1186/s13019-021-01485-z

Nakada T, Ohtsuka T (2023) Thoracic drain management using a digital system. J Thorac Dis 15(2):219. https://doi.org/10.21037/jtd-22-1692

Piler T, Schauer M, Larisch C, Riedel J, Neu R, Hofmann HS, Ried M (2024) Priorities and strategy for the implementation of enhanced recovery after surgery (ERAS) in thoracic surgery. J Thorac Dis 16(7):4165. https://doi.org/10.21037/jtd-23-1866

Sorino C, Feller-Kopman D, Mei F, Mondoni M, Agati S, Marchetti G, Rahman NM (2024) Chest tubes and pleural drainage: history and current status in pleural disease management. J Clin Med 13(21):6331. https://doi.org/10.3390/jcm13216331

St-Onge S, Chauvette V, Hamad R, Bouchard D, Jeanmart H, Lamarche Y, Perrault LP, Demers P (2021) Active clearance vs conventional management of chest tubes after cardiac surgery: a randomized controlled study. J Cardiothorac Surg 16:1–9. https://doi.org/10.1186/s13019-021-01414-0

Walcott-Sapp S, Sukumar M (2015) A history of thoracic drainage: from ancient Greeks to wound sucking drummers to digital monitoring. CTSNet. April 9, 2015. Available online: https://www.ctsnet.org/article/history-thoracic-drainage-ancient-greeks-wound-sucking-drummers-digital-monitoring. Accessed on 20 July 2025

Wang H, Hu W, Ma L, Zhang Y (2019) Digital chest drainage system versus traditional chest drainage system after pulmonary resection: a systematic review and meta-analysis. J Cardiothorac Surg 14:1–6. https://doi.org/10.1186/s13019-019-0842-x

Williams, J. G., & Lerner, A. D. (2021). Managing complications of pleural procedures. J Thorac Dis, 13(8), 5242. https://doi.org/10.21037/jtd-2019-ipicu-04

Zhou L, Guo K, Shang X, E F, Xu M, Wu Y, Yang K, Li X (2023) Advantages of applying digital chest drainage system for postoperative management of patients following pulmonary resection: a systematic review and meta-analysis of 12 randomized controlled trials. Gen Thorac Cardiovasc Surg 71(1):1–11. https://doi.org/10.1007/s11748-022-01875-7

Zisis C, Tsirgogianni K, Lazaridis G, Lampaki S, Baka S, Mpoukovinas I, Karavasilis V, Kioumis I, Pitsiou G, Katsikogiannis N, Tsakiridis K, Rapti A, Trakada G, Karapantzos I, Karapantzou C, Zissimopoulos A, Zarogoulidis K, Zarogoulidis P (2015) Chest drainage systems in use. Ann Transl Med 3(3):43. https://doi.org/10.3978/j.issn.2305-5839.2015.02.09

Enhancing Quality of Life Through Enterostomal Therapy Nursing (Stoma Care Nursing): Challenges and Solutions

14

Wai-Kuen Michelle Lee, Alice Yip, Jeff Yip, and Zoe Tsui

Introduction

Enterostomal Therapy Nursing (Stoma Care Nursing), a subspecialty within nursing practice, has historically been marginalized and often perceived negatively by healthcare professionals, who may find its clinical aspects challenging or undesirable (Hibbert 2021). Similarly, from the patients' perspective, fecal or urinary ostomies can be profoundly distressing (Assmann et al. 2024; Mohamed et al. 2021). The uncontrolled elimination of excreta through the abdominal wall presents not only physiological challenges, such as skin complications, but also significant psychosocial burdens, including fear, embarrassment, and social isolation. Moreover, the uncertainty surrounding their future health status can contribute to psychological distress (Assmann et al. 2024; Mohamed et al. 2021). Negative attitudes or lack of understanding from family and social networks may exacerbate this stress, potentially amplifying patients' anxiety and concerns. Effective stoma management, coupled with comprehensive counseling and supportive care interventions, are essential for facilitating patient adaptation to the ostomy, mitigating psychological distress, and ultimately, enhancing their QoL (Assmann et al. 2024).

W.-K. M. Lee (✉) · A. Yip · Z. Tsui
S.K. Yee School of Health Sciences, Saint Francis University,
Tseung Kwan O, HKSAR, China
e-mail: wklee@sfu.edu.hk; khyip@sfu.edu.hk; ztsui@sfu.edu.hk

J. Yip
Tung Wah College, Ho Man Tin, HKSAR, China
e-mail: jeffreyyip@twc.edu.hk

Evolution of Enterostomal Therapy Nursing (Stoma Care Nursing)

The earliest documented account of a surgically created intestinal ostomy dates to the early 1700s (Lawrence 2018; Richardson 1973). German surgeon Lorenz Heister described the externalization of a wounded soldier's intestine through the abdominal wall, a procedure now recognized as an enterostomy (Tebala 2015). However, detailed records regarding the specific care provided to these patients remain absent from the literature until the late 1930s (Elcoat 1986; Wu 2011). During this period, individuals with ostomies lacked access to specialized professional care. Consequently, they relied on resourcefulness and self-care strategies, often sharing advice and support within patient networks to address their unique challenges.

Norma Gill

Enterostomal therapy nursing owes its evolution significantly to the vision of two key figures: Dr. Rupert Turnbull, of the Cleveland Clinic, and Norma N. Gill, a former ostomy patient (Houston 2024). These individuals are respectively acknowledged as the Father and Mother of Enterostomal Therapy (Martin and Vogel 2012).

Norma Gill, considered the first stoma therapist, did not have formal nursing training. She was a patient who had undergone an ileostomy. In 1958, Dr. Rupert Turnbull recruited Gill to assist in the rehabilitation of new ostomy patients at the Cleveland Clinic (Elcoat 1986). Recognizing the growing need for specialized care for ostomy patients, both believed that a dedicated program should be implemented for individuals who had undergone ostomy surgery. In 1961, the first formal training program for stoma care was established at the Cleveland Clinic, and the term "enterostomal therapist (ET)" was coined. By the 1970s, the importance of enterostomal therapy as a specialized nursing field gained international recognition. In 1978, Norma Gill, along with other international pioneers in the field, founded the World Council of Enterostomal Therapists (WCET), a global organization for ETs (WCET® 2025).

Over the years, numerous recognized ET programs have been established internationally, and the role of the ET has expanded to include wound and continence care. Although the WCET® retains its historic designation of ET, its members' scope of practice now includes stoma, wound, and continence care.

Hong Kong

In Hong Kong, prior to the 1970s, knowledge and skills in stoma care nursing were limited. Similar to other countries, ostomy patients often relied on their own resourcefulness for stoma management. Healthcare professionals, particularly nurses, could offer only limited information. Furthermore, these patients frequently experienced neglect due to societal discrimination (Wang et al. 2022). In 1980, the first stoma care services were initiated at Queen Mary Hospital on a voluntary basis. By 1982, the first structured stoma care clinic was established at Tang Chi Ngong Clinic under the Department of Surgery of Queen Mary Hospital. This clinic provided ostomy patients with formal access to expert advice on stoma care and the management of stomal and peristomal skin complications. Subsequently, the service expanded significantly throughout various clusters of the Hospital Authority during the 1990s.

Role of Enterostomal Therapists (Stoma Care Nurse)

Clinician

Within the field of ET nursing, counseling is of most, particularly for patients with ostomies. Many individuals who undergo ostomy surgery experience a range of psychological challenges, including alterations in body images, diminished self-esteem, negative self-concept, denial, and phantom rectum sensations (Tonks 2023). These psychological results can contribute to depression, social isolation, and even suicidal ideation (Alenezi et al. 2021; Liao et al. 2024). Preoperative counseling and education regarding the alteration of elimination patterns, specifically the diversion of fecal matter through the abdomen into an ostomy pouch, are crucial for both patients and their families (Tonks 2023). Multiple sessions may be necessary to ensure patients' psychological preparedness and acceptance of ostomy surgery. Continued follow-up care is essential, even after discharge, as emotional challenges can persist for months or even years. ET nurses play a crucial role in providing specialized care, including the selection and application of appropriate ostomy appliances for various types of ostomies (Panattoni et al. 2023). They are also instrumental in the early detection and management of stomal and peristomal complications, as well as a range of wound and continence issues.

Consultation

ET nurses also serve as valuable resource persons, providing information on community resources, relevant agencies, and various products related to ostomy care, wound management, and continence (Panattoni et al. 2023). Access to comprehensive information empowers patients and their families to make informed decisions regarding their specific needs and challenges (Yip et al. 2021). Adequate preparation, including access to necessary products, facilitates a smoother transition from hospital to community settings. This in turn, promotes patients' adaptation and enables them to resume their previous lifestyles more effectively (Panattoni et al. 2023).

Liaison

Effective communication across all levels of care is fundamental to optimal patient outcomes. ET nurses serve as a vital liaison between healthcare team members, agencies, community resources, families, and patients, fostering collaboration and adherence to the established treatment plan (Panattoni et al. 2023).

Education

Patient and family education is paramount in this specialized nursing field. Instruction regarding stoma care and adaptation to life with an ostomy is crucial for successful rehabilitation. To enhance the quality of care, both classroom and clinical instruction are essential for disseminating the requisite knowledge and skills to nursing staff (Panattoni et al. 2023).

Research

Contemporary nursing practice should be grounded in evidence-based research (Nelson-Brantley and Chipps 2021). To optimize patient care, ET nurses actively participate in research studies that contribute to the development of new appliances, products, equipment, and techniques within the field of ET nursing (Keng et al. 2021).

Management

Effective functioning requires ET nurses to participate in resource planning, including developing business plans for service development and managing budgets for personnel, equipment, and consumables (Panattoni et al. 2023). Furthermore, they are involved in coordinating staffing and specialized services for in-patients, outpatient clinics, and home healthcare provided by community nurses.

History of Stoma Care Products

While stoma surgery dates to the eighteenth century, early ostomates lacked proper appliances, relying on makeshift devices like cotton- or cloth-filled cups and tins for waste collection (Elcoat 1986) (Fig. 14.1). These offered minimal skin protection and odor control. Koenig's introduction of rubber bags in 1944 marked a significant advancement, though issues with leakage and skin irritation persisted (Fig. 14.2)

Fig. 14.1 Early home-made devices

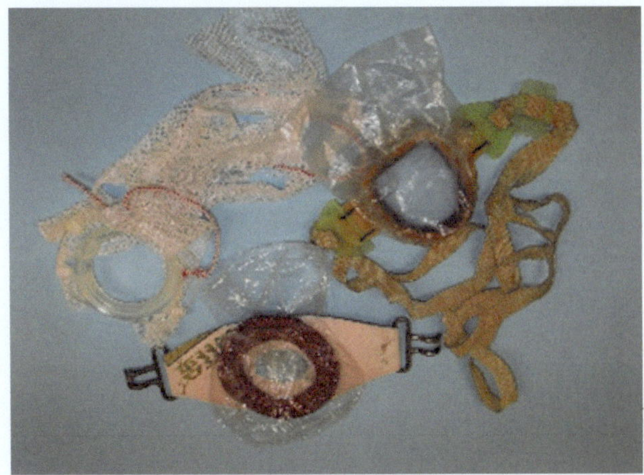

Fig. 14.2 Rubber bags

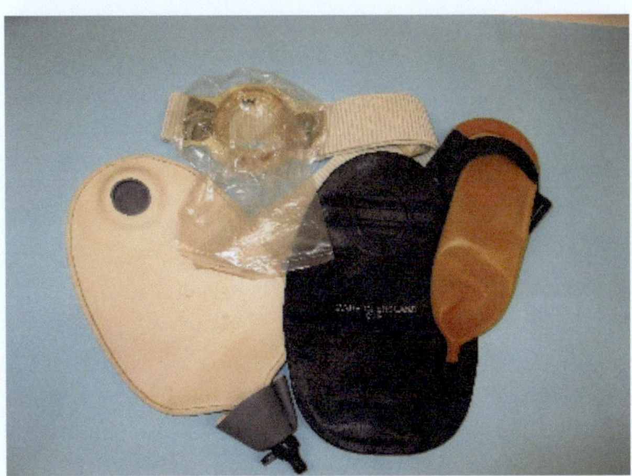

(Elcoat 1986). The 1960s brought the revolutionary development of Karaya gum and hydrocolloid skin barriers, significantly improving skin health and appliance security (Gilpin et al. 2024; Prasad et al. 2023). Concurrently, laminated plastic pouches replaced rubber bags, enhancing patient comfort.

Recent decades have witnessed dramatic improvements in stoma appliance quality. Ideal appliances feature hypoallergenic, skin-friendly, leak-proof barriers that are easy to apply and remove, coupled with quiet, discreet, and odor-proof plastic pouches (Black 2007; Elcoat 1986) (Figs. 14.3, 14.4, and 14.5). These diverse appliances accommodate various stoma types, significantly enhancing ostomates' QoL.

Fig. 14.3 Close end bag

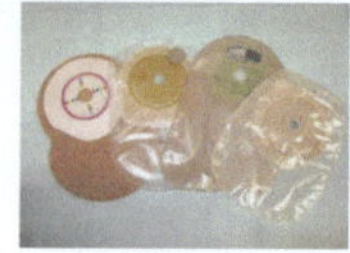

Fig. 14.4 Drainable bag

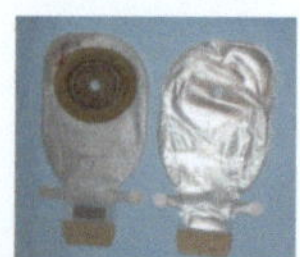

Fig. 14.5 Urostomy bag

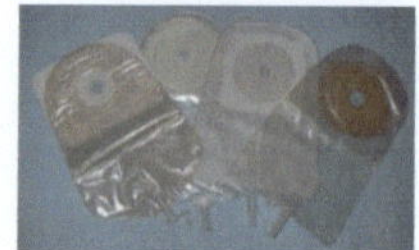

Stoma Care Products

Stoma Bags

Types	Close end bag (Fig. 14.3)	Drainable bag (Fig. 14.4)	Urostomy bag (Fig. 14.5)
Excretion	Soft to formed stool	Loose to fluid-like stool	Urine
Charcoal filter	Yes	Yes/No	No
Frequency of change	2–3 times daily	Every 2–3 days	Every 3–5 days
Special feature	Dispose once 1/3 or half full	Bottom can be opened and attached with plastic clip, soft metal tag or Velcro for secure closure. Loose to fluid-like stool can be emptied through the open bottom	Contains non-reflux valve to prevent urine reflux. With tap outlet to empty urine and connect to night-drainage bag

The appliances are available in both one-piece and two-piece systems, each incorporating a skin barrier to enhance cutaneous protection (Harris 2021; Rolfsen et al. 2024). Ostomy bags are provided with either precut or customizable skin barriers to accommodate varying patient requirements. Furthermore, convex skin barriers have been developed to address retracted stomas (Fig. 14.6), a condition often associated with leakage and subsequent skin excoriation. The convex design applies gentle pressure to the peristomal skin, thereby promoting stoma protrusion and mitigating the risk of leakage.

Fig. 14.6 Ostomy bags with convex skin barriers

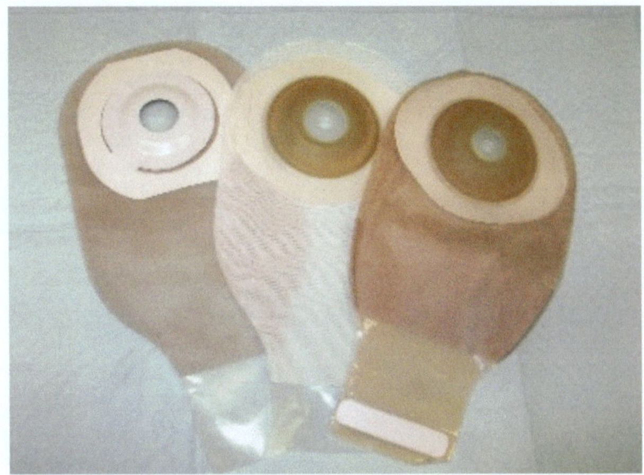

Fig. 14.7 Seals

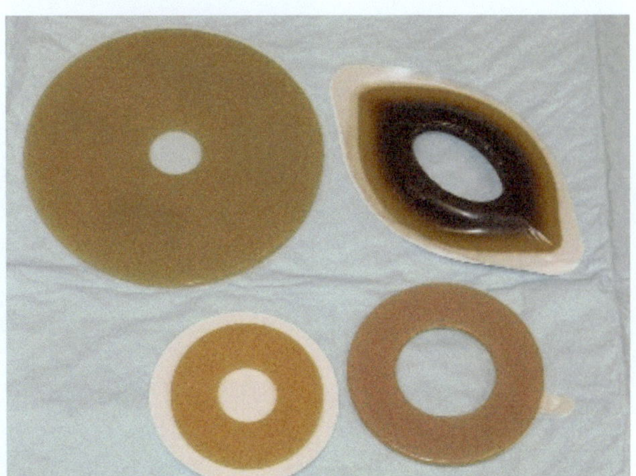

Stoma Accessories

Stoma accessories	Features
Skin protective barrier/wafer/sheet	It is the combination of adhesive materials, polymeric matrices and sodium carboxymethylcellulose to promote healing of large excoriated peristomal areas
Protective powder	Absorbs moisture, promoting wound healing on reddened, sore, or broken peristomal skin
Paste	Stoma paste fills creases, creating a smooth surface for appliance or skin barrier attachment
Seals (Fig. 14.7)	Alcohol-free, absorbent stoma seals (sodium carboxymethylcellulose) mold and fill skin dips, creating a smooth surface for adhesives
Adhesive remover	Adhesive removers (alcohol, oil, or silicone-based) aid in appliance and residue removal

(continued)

Stoma accessories	Features
Protective film	Skin barrier film enhance adhesion, extending wear time of stoma appliances
Skin cleanser	Skin wipes clean the area around the stoma for pouch changes
Flatus filter	Charcoal filters in ostomy pouches vent gas and control odour
Deodorant	Deodorant (spray, powder, drops) masks or neutralizes ostomy odour
Ostomy belt	Elastic belts enhance the security of ostomy appliances
Protective shield (Fig. 14.8)	Plastic stoma guards protect the stoma during sport activities
Stoma cap (Fig. 14.9)	Small, low-capacity pouches cover colostomies after irrigation or for swimming

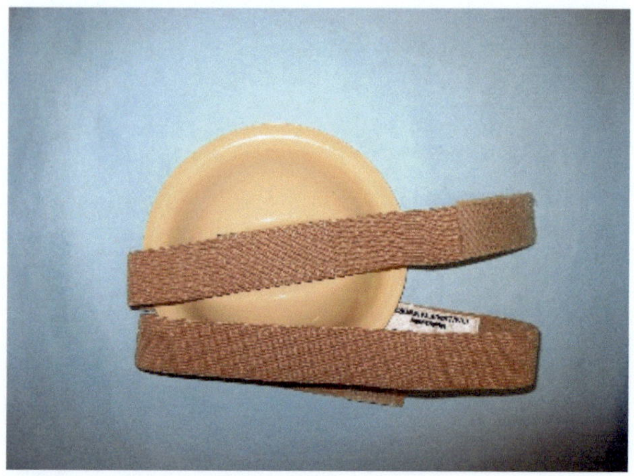

Fig. 14.8 Protective shield

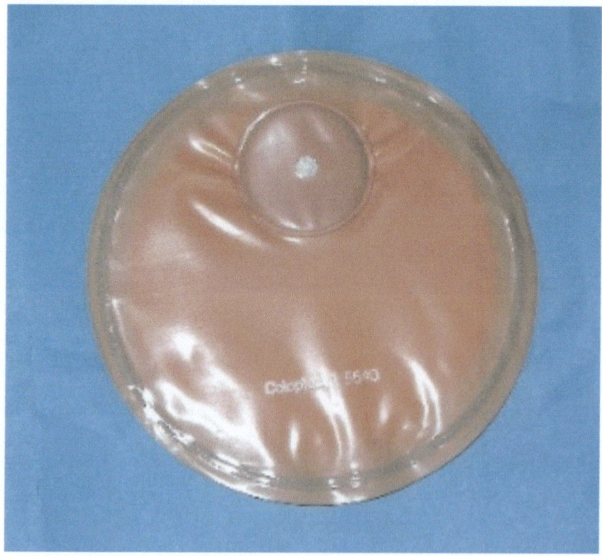

Fig. 14.9 Stoma cap

Common Complications Related to Stoma and Peristomal Skin

Ostomy complications can be physiological (e.g., constipation, high output, electrolyte imbalances), psychological (e.g., body image issues, depression), or physical (e.g., skin irritation, sexual problems) (Black and Notter 2021; Duque et al. 2023). This chapter discusses physical stoma complications, manageable through surgery, medication, adjusted stoma care, or specialized products. These include stoma and peristomal complications.

Stoma Complications

Ischemia

A healthy stoma presents as warm, moist, and red. Ischemia, resulting from comprising blood supply (Fig. 14.10), can occur due to mesenteric tension, vessel ligation, or excessive mesenteric dissection (Babakhanlou et al. 2022). It may also arise from appliance or clothing constriction (Ambe et al. 2018). Ischemia compromises stoma viability and necessitates prompt surgical consultation. A dusky stoma warrants close monitoring. Progression to black signifies complete vascular compromise and eventual necrosis, requiring timely stoma revision (Murken and Bleier 2019; Tsujinaka et al. 2020).

Problems Encountered

Lacking sensation, patients are often unaware of stomal ischemia until necrosis occurs. Complete necrosis can lead to detachment, retraction below the fascia, and subsequent peritoneal contamination or infection.

Fig. 14.10 Ischemia of the stoma

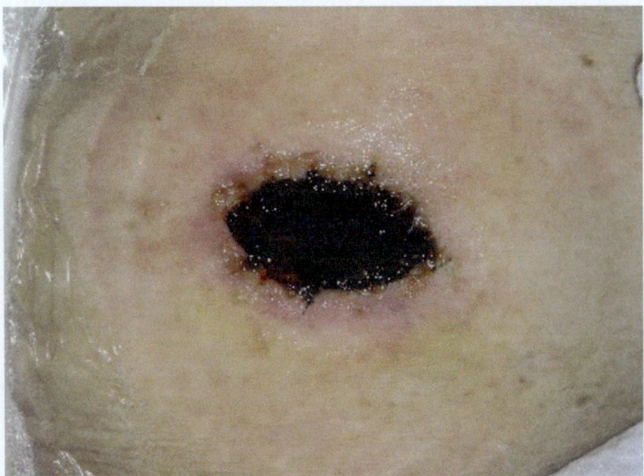

Intervention

To prevent constriction from postoperative swelling, the initial appliance should be slightly larger than the stoma. A transparent appliance facilitates stomal color monitoring. Color changes constitute a surgical emergency requiring immediate consultation.

Superficial ischemia, typically confined to the stomal mucosa, often resolves spontaneously with sloughing of the affected area, leaving a healthy stoma. However, long-term complications, such as retraction or stenosis, potentially leading to leakage (Murken and Bleier 2019; Tsujinaka et al. 2020), may occur. Ischemia extending below the fascia necessitates surgical debridement and stoma reconstruction (Babakhanlou et al. 2022). Regardless of severity, providing reassurance and thorough explanations to patients is crucial for alleviating anxiety.

Stenosis

Stomal stenosis, a narrowing of the stomal outlet at either the fascial or cutaneous level (Fig. 14.11), can cause partial or complete obstruction of fecal flow (Krishnamurty et al. 2017). Contributing factors include scarring, surgical technique, infection, mucocutaneous separation, and ischemia (Babakhanlou et al. 2022; Stelton 2019).

Problems Encountered

In fecal stomas, stenosis can cause pain during defecation or even bowel obstruction (Krishnamurty et al. 2017). In urostomies, stenosis may lead to recurrent urinary tract infections.

Intervention

Ostomates should be advised to use mild laxatives and increase fluid intake to prevent bowel obstruction. Symptoms, like nausea, vomiting, decreased output, distension, pain, and cramping, warrant immediate medical attention (Babakhanlou et al. 2022). Cutaneous stenosis can be managed with local revision (Ambe et al. 2022). Fascial stenosis may benefit from careful digital dilation or use of a stoma dilator,

Fig. 14.11 Stomal stenosis

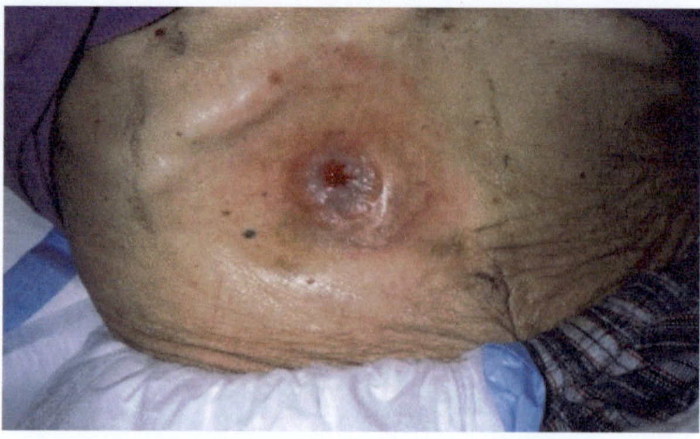

Fig. 14.12 Stomal retraction

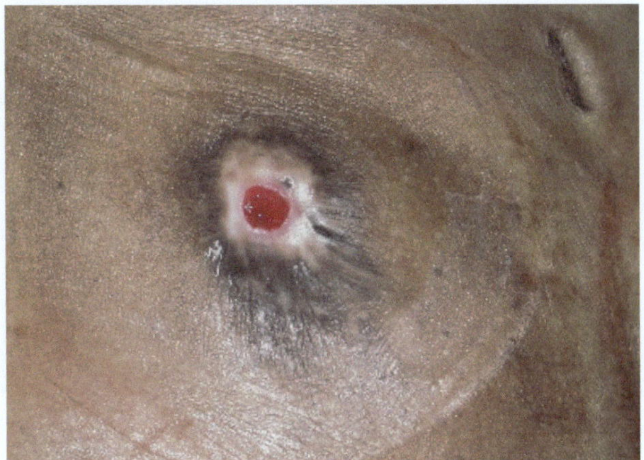

though excessive force can exacerbate scarring (Stelton 2019). Severe stenosis often requires surgical refashioning.

Retraction

Stomal retraction, a recession of the stoma (Fig. 14.12), can result from inadequate mobilization or fixation, premature rod removal, weight gain, necrosis, or mucocutaneous separation (Krishnamurty et al. 2017).

Problems Encountered

Retraction hinders appliance adhesion, causing leakage, skin irritation, and psychological stress.

Intervention

Mild retraction can be managed with seals, paste, convex appliances, and belts (Ambe et al. 2022; Stelton 2019). Skin protectants address excoriation. Weight loss may help if retraction is due to postoperative weight gain. Severe, persistent leakage necessitates surgical revision.

Prolapse

Prolapse, common in loop colostomies (incidence ~30%), occurs when the bowel protrudes through the stoma (Fig. 14.13) (Krishnamurty et al. 2017; Tsujinaka et al. 2020). Causes include inadequate stomal fixation, obesity, and increased abdominal pressure (Babakhanlou et al. 2022).

Problems Encountered

Prolapse causes pain, appliance fitting difficulties, and potential trauma (ulceration, bleeding) during bag changes (Babakhanlou et al. 2022). Edema and friction from the appliance increase trauma risk, and ischemia may result due to stoma constriction by the appliance. Kinking of the prolapsed bowel may cause strangulation and obstruction. The protruding bowel also impacts psychological well-being, causing

Fig. 14.13 Prolapse

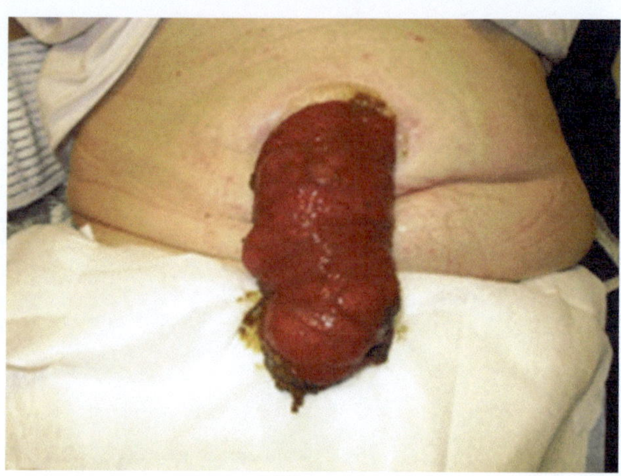

anxiety and distress due to its appearance and detectability under clothing (Ambe et al. 2022).

Intervention

A large-opening appliance minimizes friction, trauma, and constriction of the prolapsed bowel. Patients should monitor stoma color and report signs of bowel obstruction immediately, as these require emergency management. Mild prolapse can be manually reduced with the patient lying flat, using cold compresses or sugar powder to reduce edema (Ambe et al. 2022; Krishnamurty et al. 2017). A stoma shield can help maintain reduction. Severe or complicated prolapse (e.g., ischemia) requires surgical intervention.

Peristomal Complications

Allergy

Allergic contact dermatitis is skin inflammation caused by allergy to stoma care products (Stelton 2019). Symptoms include redness, blisters, weeping, itching, and a rash mirroring the adhesive or bag shape (Fig. 14.14) (Stelton 2019). Severe reaction can spread beyond the initial contact area.

Problems Encountered

Weeping skin and blisters can prevent proper appliance adhesion, causing leaks and worsening skin problem.

Intervention

Identify and remove the allergy-causing substance. Try alternative appliances with different adhesives or wafers. Eliminate potential irritants (paste, remover, etc.) one by one. If the allergen remains unknown, consult a dermatologist for patch testing.

Fig. 14.14 Allergy

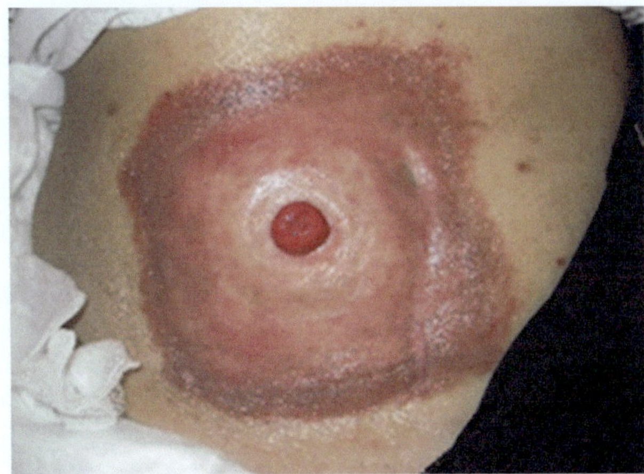

Fig. 14.15 Peristomal skin redness and ulceration

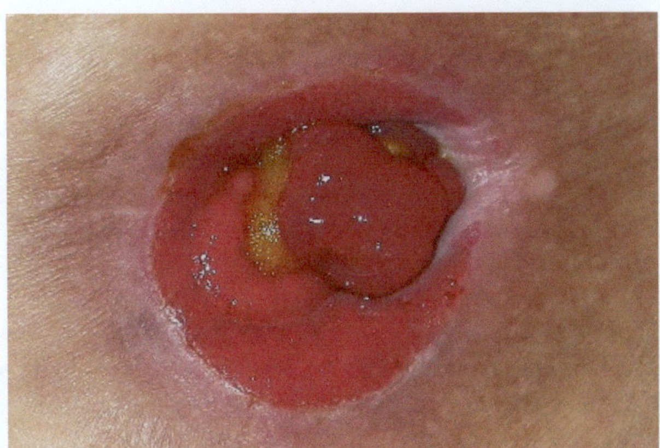

Applying short-term corticosteroid ointment helps suppress the local immune response (Stelton 2019; Mijaljica et al. 2022). Ensure it dries completely before applying a skin barrier. Protective powder can absorb moisture, improving adhesion.

Effluent Dermatitis

Prolonged contact with stoma output (feces or urine) can cause peristomal skin redness and ulceration (Fig. 14.15) (O'Flynn 2019; Stelton 2019). This is most common with ileostomies due to corrosive enzymes and electrolytes in the output (Brzezinski 2024; Williams and Carlson 2023). Longer contact leads to greater damage, progressing from irritation to denuded skin. Common causes include leaving the appliance on too long, leakage between the barrier and skin, and an overly large barrier opening.

Problems Encountered

Excoriated skin becomes painful, even with gentle cleansing, causing stress with each pouch change. Sore skin hinders appliance adhesion, leading to more leakage and worsening skin problems.

Intervention

Identify the cause of effluent dermatitis: uneven skin, deep creases, stoma retraction, or a large barrier opening. Cleanse sore skin gently with warm water and apply protective powder. A layer of non-alcohol protective film after powder application may also help in some situations. Use seals for creases and alcohol-free paste around the barrier opening to prevent leakage. A convex barrier can help with retracted stomas. An ostomy belt adds security. Ensure the barrier opening is appropriately sized to protect the skin from effluent.

Parastomal Hernia

A parastomal hernia is an incisional hernia adjacent to a stoma, where a loop of intestine protrudes through a weakened abdominal wall (Ishimaru et al. 2021; Zhu et al. 2024). Risk factors include age, gender, body mass index, previous surgery, chronic illnesses (e.g., diabetes, COPD), subcutaneous fat thickness, stoma type, stoma placement (away from the rectus abdominis), surgical approach (open vs. laparoscopic), and incision complications (Manole et al. 2023; Zhu et al. 2024). Bulging can range from slight to large (Fig. 14.16). The incidence is likely underestimated, with reported prevalence between 30% and 50% (Manole et al. 2023).

Problems Encountered

The hernia's shape can obscure the stoma, making appliance application difficult and leading to leakage (Babakhanlou et al. 2022). The bulge can cause discomfort, altered bowel habits, dragging sensations, and embarrassment, potentially impacting body image and causing anxiety. Bowel kinking or strangulation within the hernia can lead

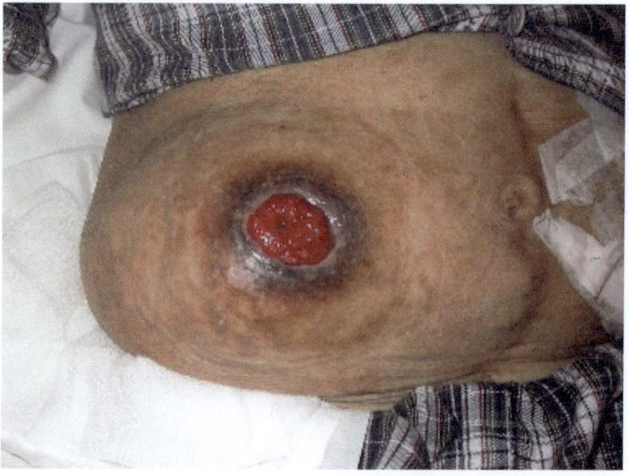

Fig. 14.16 Parastomal hernia

to obstruction, requiring surgery or causing life-threatening complications. These symptoms significantly affect the patient's QoL (Murken and Bleier 2019).

Intervention

Ostomates with hernia may need a more flexible appliance and accessories, like paste, seals, wipes, or a belt for secure fixation. If the stoma is obscured, using a mirror during pouch changes may be necessary. Colostomy irrigation may become ineffective, and resuming natural evacuation might be recommended (Stelton 2019). Hernia support garments can reduce dragging sensations, improve comfort, and conceal the hernia. Educate ostomates about emergency signs of bowel strangulation (abdominal pain, absent stoma output, vomiting, stoma color change), requiring immediate medical attention (Babakhanlou et al. 2022).

Enhancing Client QoL: Key Contributions

Stoma formation presents significant life challenges. Multiple studies demonstrated how stomas can be stigmatizing, leading to feelings of disability (Kittscha et al. 2022; Xian et al. 2018). Changes in body image, elimination processes, religious and cultural beliefs, lifestyle, and sexuality all impact ostomates' adaptation. This can result in low self-esteem, anxiety, depression, social isolation, hopelessness, and even suicidal thoughts (Sarabi 2020; Yip et al. 2021). Greater stoma acceptance correlates with better psychological adjustment, rehabilitation, and QoL (Kittscha et al. 2022; Zhang et al. 2019). Reducing negativity, promoting independence, encouraging social interaction, and facilitating a return to normal life are crucial for improving well-being and reducing feelings of hopelessness and suicidal ideation.

Long-term care, providing close monitoring and continuous psychosocial support, is crucial for patient rehabilitation (Smith and Cook 2024). ETs play a key role beyond physical and client education. They provide early detection and management of stoma-related complications and skin problems, ensuring smooth transitions from hospital to community, preventing readmissions, and addressing psychological needs. ETs require advanced education, clinical competence, experience, and critical thinking to improve ostomates' QoL (NHS Education for Scotland 2021). Despite their vital contributions, ETs are often undervalued (Rolls et al. 2024). Greater recognition of this specialty will benefit more ostomates (Bird et al. 2023; Rolls et al. 2024).

Conclusion

Stoma formation, while often lifesaving, can cause significant physical and psychological trauma. Although some patients adapt well over time, others struggle to adjust. Many factors influence their coping process. Continuous support from a multidisciplinary healthcare team, family, and society is crucial. With appropriate support and guidance, these patients can achieve a good QoL despite the challenges.

References

Alenezi A, McGrath I, Kimpton A, Livesay K (2021) Quality of life among ostomy patients: a narrative literature review. J Clin Nurs 30(21–22):3111–3123. https://doi.org/10.1111/jocn.15840

Ambe PC, Kurz NR, Nitschke C, Odeh SF, Möslein G, Zirngibl H (2018) Intestinal ostomy: classification, indications, ostomy care and complication management. Dtsch Arztebl Int 115(11):182. https://doi.org/10.3238/arztebl.2018.0182

Ambe PC, Kugler CM, Breuing J, Grohmann E, Friedel J, Hess S, Pieper D (2022) The effect of preoperative stoma site marking on risk of stoma-related complications in patients with intestinal ostomy—a systematic review and meta-analysis. Color Dis 24(8):904–917. https://doi.org/10.1111/codi.16118

Assmann SL, Keszthelyi D, Breukink SO, Kimman ML (2024) Living with faecal incontinence: a qualitative investigation of patient experiences and preferred outcomes through semi-structured interviews. Qual Life Res:1–9. https://doi.org/10.1007/s11136-024-03756-3

Babakhanlou R, Larkin K, Hita AG, Stroh J, Yeung SC (2022) Stoma-related complications and emergencies. Int J Emerg Med 15(1):17. https://doi.org/10.1186/s12245-022-00421-9

Bird A, Burch J, Thorpe G (2023) The role of the clinical nurse specialist in stoma care: a scoping review. Br J Nurs 32(16):S6–S16. https://doi.org/10.12968/bjon.2023.32.16.S6

Black P (2007) Peristomal skin care: an overview of available products. Br J Nurs 16(17):1048–1056. https://doi.org/10.12968/bjon.2007.16.17.27249

Black P, Notter J (2021) Psychological issues affecting patients living with a stoma. Br J Nurs 30(6):S20–S32. https://doi.org/10.12968/bjon.2021.30.6.S20

Brzezinski A (2024) Medical management of the patient with an ostomy. In: Crohn's disease. CRC Press, pp 417–423

Duque PA, Valencia Rico CL, Campiño Valderrama SM, López González LA (2023) Effects of socio-educational interventions on the quality of life of people with a digestive ostomy. SAGE Open Nurs 9:23779608231177542. https://doi.org/10.1177/23779608231177542

Elcoat C (1986) Stoma care nursing. Bailliere Tindall, London

Gilpin V, Magee N, Scott C, Pourshahidi LK, Gill CI, Simpson EE, McCreadie K, Davis J (2024) Evolution of ostomy pouch design: opportunities for composite technologies to advance patient care. J Compos Sci 8(10):388. https://doi.org/10.3390/jcs8100388

Harris G (2021) Stoma care appliances: an overview. Gastrointest Nurs 19(Sup9):S14–S19. https://doi.org/10.12968/gasn.2021.19.Sup9.S14

Hibbert D (2021) The role and practice of clinical nurse specialists: an international focus on Saudi Arabia. In: Clinical nurse specialist role and practice: an international perspective. Springer International Publishing, Cham, pp 213–223

Houston N (2024) Norma N Gill: a symphony of resilience and reform in enterostomal therapy. World Council Enteros Ther J 44(1):40–48

Ishimaru K, Shuno Y, Nozawa H, Kawai K, Murono K, Ishihara S (2021) Risk factors for parastomal hernia associated with covering stoma in rectal surgery. Indian J Surg 83(Suppl 3):749–754. https://doi.org/10.1007/s12262-021-02803-4

Keng CJ, Lee J, Valencia M, McKechnie T, Forbes S, Eskicioglu C (2021) Transition home following new fecal ostomy creation: a qualitative study. J Wound Ostomy Cont Nurs 48(6):537–543. https://doi.org/10.1097/WON.0000000000000814

Kittscha J, Fairbrother G, Bliokas V, Wilson V (2022) Adjustment to an ostomy: an integrative literature review. J Wound Ostomy Cont Nurs 49(5):439–448. https://doi.org/10.1097/WON.0000000000000895

Krishnamurty DM, Blatnik J, Mutch M (2017) Stoma complications. Clin Colon Rectal Surg 30(03):193–200. https://doi.org/10.1055/s-0037-1598160

Lawrence C (ed) (2018) Medical theory, surgical practice: studies in the history of surgery. Routledge, Abingdon

Liao Y, Liu X, Wu X, Li C, Li Y (2024) Social isolation profiles and conditional process analysis among postoperative enterostomy patients with colorectal cancer. BMC Psychol 12(1):782. https://doi.org/10.1186/s40359-024-02304-5

Manole TE, Daniel I, Alexandra B, Dan PN, Andronic O (2023) Risk factors for the development of parastomal hernia: a narrative review. Saudi J Med Med Sci 11(3):187–192. https://doi.org/10.4103/sjmms.sjmms_235_22

Martin ST, Vogel JD (2012) Intestinal stomas: indications, management, and complications. Adv Surg 46(1):19–49. https://doi.org/10.1016/j.yasu.2012.04.005

Mijaljica D, Spada F, Harrison IP (2022) Emerging trends in the use of topical antifungal-corticosteroid combinations. J Fungi 8(8):812. https://doi.org/10.3390/jof8080812

Mohamed NE, Shah QN, Kata HE, Sfakianos J, Given B (2021, February) Dealing with the unthinkable: bladder and colorectal cancer patients' and informal caregivers' unmet needs and challenges in life after ostomies. In: Seminars in oncology nursing, Vol. 37, No. 1. WB Saunders, p 151111. https://doi.org/10.1016/j.soncn.2020.151111

Murken DR, Bleier JI (2019) Ostomy-related complications. Clin Colon Rectal Surg 32(03):176–182. https://doi.org/10.1055/s-0038-1676995

Nelson-Brantley HV, Chipps E (2021) Implementation science and nursing leadership: improving the adoption and sustainability of evidence-based practice. J Nurs Adm 51(5):237–239. https://doi.org/10.1097/NNA.0000000000001006

NHS Education for Scotland (2021) Advanced nursing practice (ANP). Online available: https://www.nes.scot.nhs.uk/our-work/advanced-nursing-practice-anp/. Accessed on 30 June 2025

O'Flynn SK (2019) Peristomal skin damage: assessment, prevention and treatment. Br J Nurs 28(5):S6–S12. https://doi.org/10.12968/bjon.2019.28.5.S6

Panattoni N, Mariani R, Spano A, Leo AD, Iacorossi L, Petrone F, Simone ED (2023) Nurse specialist and ostomy patient: competence and skills in the care pathway. A scoping review. J Clin Nurs 32(17–18):5959–5973. https://doi.org/10.1111/jocn.16722

Prasad N, Thombare N, Sharma SC, Kumar S (2023) Recent development in the medical and industrial applications of gum karaya: a review. Polym Bull 80(4):3425–3447. https://doi.org/10.1007/s00289-022-04227-w

Richardson RG (1973) The abdominable stoma: a historical survey of the artificial anus. Abbott Laboratories, pp 1–56

Rolfsen T, Vestergaard M, Hansen MF, Boisen EB, Dambæk MR (2024) Body fit with a pouching system with concave contour for people with an outward peristomal body profile: effects on leakage, wear time, and quality of life: a randomized controlled cross-over trial. J Wound Ostomy Cont Nurs 51(4):303–311. https://doi.org/10.1097/WON.0000000000001088

Rolls N, Carvalho F, Hall A, Osborne W (2024) Raising the voice of specialist stoma care nurses: a call for a national strategy in stoma care. Br J Nurs 33(16):S4–S12. https://doi.org/10.12968/bjon.2024.0074

Sarabi N (2020) Hopelessness and suicide ideation in ostomy patients: a mixed method study. J Coloproctol 40(3):214–219. https://doi.org/10.1016/j.jcol.2020.05.008

Smith C, Cook N (2024) Ostomy care nurses' knowledge and practice related to prevention and management of parastomal hernias in adults: a nationwide survey of UK stoma care nurses. J Wound Ostomy Cont Nurs 51(4):289–296. https://doi.org/10.1097/WON.0000000000001091

Stelton S (2019) CE: stoma and peristomal skin care: a clinical review. Am J Nurs 119(6):38–45. https://doi.org/10.1097/01.NAJ.0000559781.86311.64

Tebala GD (2015) History of colorectal surgery: a comprehensive historical review from the ancient Egyptians to the surgical robot. Int J Color Dis 30:723–748. https://doi.org/10.1007/s00384-015-2152-7

Tonks N (2023) Body image and sexuality. In: Stoma care specialist nursing: a guide for clinical practice. Springer International Publishing, Cham, pp 287–299. https://doi.org/10.1007/978-3-031-07799-9_16

Tsujinaka S, Tan KY, Miyakura Y, Fukano R, Oshima M, Konishi F, Rikiyama T (2020) Current management of intestinal stomas and their complications. J Anus Rectum Colon 4(1):25–33. https://doi.org/10.23922/jarc.2019-032

Wang Y, Li S, Gong J, Cao L, Xu D, Yu Q, Wang X, Chen Y (2022) Perceived stigma and self-efficacy of patients with inflammatory bowel disease-related stoma in China: a cross-sectional study. Front Med 9:813367. https://doi.org/10.3389/fmed.2022.813367

Williams, L., & Carlson, G. L. (2023). Care of Intestinal Stoma and Enterocutaneous Fistula (s). In Intestinal Failure (pp. 619-630). Cham: Springer International Publishing. https://doi.org/10.1007/978-3-031-22265-8_38

World Council of Enterostomal Therapists® (2025) Founding of the WCET. Online available: https://wcetn.org/page/History#:~:text=The%20WCET%C2%AE%20was%20formally%20founded%20on%20May%2018%2C,in%20conjunction%20with%20the%20International%20Ostomy%20Association%20%28IOA%29. Accessed on 30 July 2025

Wu JS (2011) Intestinal stomas: historical overview. In: Atlas of intestinal stomas. Springer US, Boston, pp 1–37

Xian H, Zhang Y, Yang Y, Zhang X, Wang X (2018) A descriptive, cross-sectional study among Chinese patients to identify factors that affect psychosocial adjustment to an enterostomy. Ostomy Wound Manage 64(7):8–17. https://doi.org/10.25270/owm.2018.7.817

Yip YC, Tsui WK, Yip KH (2021) Hong Kong's growing need for palliative care services and the role of the nursing profession. Asia Pac J Health Manag 16(1):i597, 1–7. https://doi.org/10.24083/apjhm.v16i1.597

Zhang Y, Xian H, Yang Y, Zhang X, Wang X (2019) Relationship between psychosocial adaptation and health-related quality of life of patients with stoma: a descriptive, cross-sectional study. J Clin Nurs 28(15–16):2880–2888. https://doi.org/10.1111/jocn.14876

Zhu L, Li S, Wang F (2024) Risk factors for parastomal hernia after abdominoperineal resection of rectal cancer. Front Oncol 14:1470113. https://doi.org/10.3389/fonc.2024.1470113

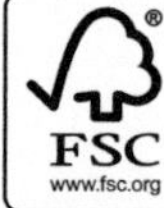